You Are Not Alone
Real World Solutions for Family Caregivers

You Are Not Alone
Real World Solutions for Family Caregivers

GARY EDWARD BARG
Editor-in-Chief, *Today's Caregiver* magazine

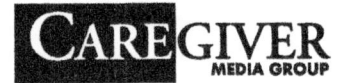

First paperback edition 2020

Copyright© 2020 by Caregiver.com, Inc.

All rights reserved. No part of this book may be reproduced or utilized in any form or by any means, electronic or mechanical, including photocopying, recording, or by any information storage and retrieval system, without permission in writing from the publisher. Inquiries should be addressed to:

Caregiver.com™
3920 Riverland Road
Fort Lauderdale, FL. 33312
www.caregiver.com

ISBN 978-0-9834066-2-4

Designed by Adnan Razack & Joshua Mesa
Cover Design by Adnan Razack & Joshua Mesa

First Edition
10 9 8 7 6 5

CONTENTS

Acknowledgments	6
Introduction	7
Chapter 1: **CARING FOR ONE ANOTHER**	23
Chapter 2: **GETTING HELP FROM OUR LOVED ONES**	57
Chapter 3: **PARTNERING WITH THE CARE TEAM**	89
Chapter 4: **EMOTIONAL SUPPORT**	113
Chapter 5: **STOP SCAMMERS**	131
Chapter 6: **YOUR LEGAL RIGHTS**	147
Chapter 7: **WORKING WITH THE SYSTEM**	175

ACKNOWLEDGMENTS

Special thanks to all of the family caregivers who have joined us at the Fearless Caregiver Conferences around the nation over these past twenty-two years for sharing their wisdom that you will find in the pages.

I would also like to thank our dedicated team of advocates and educators, Steven C. Barg, Nancy Schonwalter, Cathy Byrd, Monica Barg and Christian T. Andaya. I would also like to add my sincere appreciation to our creative team, led by Adnan D. Razack and to graphic designer Joshua Mesa.

Most important of all, thanks to you for all you do for your loved ones, friends and community in this New-New Normal world we find ourselves in the times of Covid-19.

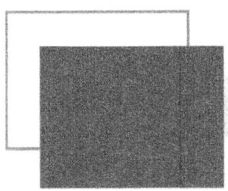

INTRODUCTION

The Fearless Caregiver Conference series began in 1998 when we wanted to bring a group of family and professional caregivers, as well as local and national advocates together for the day. The late television actor Robert Urich was the keynote speaker for that first event, having recently shared his cancer diagnosis and remission on national television. Two things were evident throughout the day, the first was that caregivers loved to share with one another and the advice they had was as effective and appropriate as any offered by the degreed professionals. And many times, much more so. The reason for this is simple. The family caregiver is the person caring for their loved one around the clock and necessarily creates solutions for the challenges that they face daily.

The other thing that was evident was that caregivers for loved ones with differing diagnoses and caregiving situations could learn from one another's experiences. I recall an interaction among four caregivers sitting around a luncheon table during that first conference. Their main care concerns were (respectively) AIDS, Parkinson's, cancer and Alzheimer's disease. As I listened in on them, they were reveling in the fact that each of them brought different but powerful experiences to the table. The caregiver whose primary care concern was AIDS talked about managing her loved ones medication regime, the Alzheimer's caregiver was sharing her challenges with the long-term care facility in which she had just placed her loved one, the cancer caregiver was discussing the clinical trial study that her loved one just joined, and the Parkinson's caregiver was talking of solutions he had come up with regarding his loved ones increasingly limited mobility. The areas of interest and the skill sets these caregivers brought to that table were both unique and of specific value to their fellow luncheon companions.

We subtitle these events "A Day of Sharing Wisdom" and these four caregivers were truly living up to the phrase. That luncheon group brought to life our concerns about the challenge of isolating and "siloing" caregivers based upon their main healthcare issues. For the longest time, caregivers were segmented by the types of disease or illness with which their loved ones were dealing. Conferences, publications and even support groups were defined by the disease and not the individual. This fact had come to life for me as I was asked to speak at a wide variety of healthcare conferences: spinal cord, Alzheimer's, Parkinson's or even scleroderma.

Certainly, the medical issues were unique to the diagnoses, but after a while the concerns and the stories of the caregivers I had met at these various events could not have been more similar. They were worried about the best care for their loved ones, had financial concerns, too much stress and too little actionable and appropriate information. Soon I became somewhat of a healthcare "Johnny Appleseed" spreading the ideas and advice I received from these different groups with the next groups I met, regardless of their loved one's disease or illness.

We took the leap on April 25th, 1998 and held our first event at Nova Southeastern University in Fort Lauderdale, Florida. There are many things we have learned since that day. No longer do we hold sessions until 5:30 p.m. like so many events. Now we call our schedule a "full caregiver's day," generally starting at 9:30 a.m. and ending at 2:30 p.m. This schedule allows for the caregivers to be able to drop their kids at school and their parents at adult day care and still have time to pick them all up at the end of the day without missing any of the conference. The other major change we made with regards to the day's schedule was to hold an open question and answer panel for all attendees in the morning session. The purpose is to have any questions posed by a caregiver in attendance answered by our panel of local and national experts. The panels have consisted of doctors, social workers, attorneys, Area Agency on Aging caregiver support professionals and even financial experts.

Once the session starts, I run around the conference room with a wireless microphone in hand as what I call a "low rent" Phil Donohue. My job is to bring some of the advice and information I learned from other caregivers in previous events held around the nation and to motivate the caregivers to interact with one another, as well as with the panel.

The secret to the success for this conference session (just between us) is that once the panel begins, the caregivers start answering each other's questions, with the experts sometimes taking notes themselves. In truth, so many times the caregivers sitting in the audience are the true experts and I know that every single professional at each event would share in this belief.

One conference remains with me to this day. The event was held at the Union League Center in downtown Philadelphia, with the remarkable Della Reese as keynote speaker. We were surrounded by original portraits of our nation's presidents hanging on the mahogany walls in this refurbished 17th century meeting house.

Towards the end of the event, a caregiver who had sat silently for most of the day raised her hand to speak. She told us that her mother was in the hospital getting prepped for surgery, but she knew that being with us was too important for her own well-being to miss. She went on to say that she was the sole informal caregiver for six of her senior neighbors and that she had two heart attacks in the past two years, as well as out of control blood pressure. As I asked her to stand and hugged her, the audience took turns giving her advice on caring for herself until a caregiver from across the room stood up and said, "I live in your neighborhood and from now on, you're not alone." Tears flowed from every eye in the room. At the next year's event, these two caregivers, now fast friends, were sitting together and told the spellbound room of their fellow caregivers of their accomplishments over the past twelve months.

Another thing about that event with Della Reese I would like to share with you is that three weeks after the event, I received an email from a family caregiver lamenting that no one in her community could or would ever understand what she was going through as a caregiver. She was convinced she was alone in her fears and concerns. The upshot of that story is that she lives not three miles from the Union League, the site of the aforementioned conference. Thankfully, she joined us at every event in her community after the one she missed.

On Becoming a Fearless Caregiver

I watched out of the corner of my eye as a conference attendee strode across the large banquet hall. She was on a mission to reach her destination and would not be deterred. And I was afraid that destination was me. The year was 2005 and I was standing in the middle of a room filled with family caregivers at one of our Fearless Caregiver Conferences. This was the 45th event that we had hosted across the country and was being held in our own hometown of Fort Lauderdale where the first event was also held in 1998.

As I mentioned before, to me the linchpin of the events is always the morning question and answer session. Frankly, it is most fun for me during these sessions when a question would arise that the panel of experts could not answer. I like to call this the "Stump the Panel" moment. Not in any way to embarrass our experts, but because I know for a fact that the other group of caregiving experts in the room will be up to the task and answer with many appropriate and innovative responses. These other experts I refer to, of course, are always family caregivers. The main reason for the exercise of answering audience questions, is to illustrate to caregivers that knowledge was not a one-way street. They (or other caregivers like them) already had more answers than they could have imagined before the questions ever started flowing in the session.

After the caregiver finally crossed the hall and reached me, she whispered in my ear as I held the microphone in front of another caregiver about to ask a question of our panel. What she whispered was this, "I have a question that I think is too stupid to ask in public and so I would like you to ask it for me." Gee, thanks. But, being her kind and humble host for the day, I quickly pointed the microphone in her direction and announced to the assemblage, "This lady has a question to ask of us." There was one reason for my action, and it had nothing to do with cruelty. For in fact, I knew that whatever question this caregiver standing before me would ask, it would be poignant, appropriate and the furthest thing from stupid.

Unfortunately, the specific question is lost in the haze of time, but I will always remember what happened next. The attorney who was serving on the question and answer panel of experts, upon hearing the question, slammed the table and said, "I've been waiting all morning for someone to ask that very question." The caregiver glided back to her seat on a cushion of air. My confidence in my actions was easy to explain; in the many years that we have been hosting the Fearless Caregiver Conferences and in the thousands of emails I have received from family caregivers since launching Today's Caregiver magazine and caregiver.com, I have never once received a silly or inappropriate question from a family caregiver. Never. This brings us to the first rule of Fearless Caregiving: Any question you have as a family caregiver is important and deserves to be answered quickly, concisely and with the respect you deserve as an equal member of your loved one's care team.

The role we caregivers play in the care of our loved ones can not easily be overstated. The average caregiver will be responsible for the directed expenditures of over $40,000 a year caring for their loved one (make it $47,000 for Alzheimer's care). They will lose over $600,000 in opportunities and promotions during the lifetime of their career and over 63% of caregivers will consider depression to be their most felt emotion. And according to a Stanford University study, nearly 40% of those of us who care for cognitively impaired loved ones will die before they do.

Then why do we do it? The answer is simple...because we can't not do it, because our loved ones need us, because we never even asked ourselves if there was any other way. Because it is who we are.

So, now what? How do we go from partner and spouse or dedicated daughter or son to becoming a dietitian, therapist, insurance specialist, immediate medical expert, chauffeur, psychologist, pharmacist and incontinence specialist? And keep our relationship with our loved ones, families, friends and neighbors, not to mention keeping our jobs, which a third of us end up losing.

I firmly believe the way that we achieve all our goals as caregivers is by taking on a new job role. That is one I call being a Fearless Caregiver. A Fearless Caregiver is a caregiver who understands that they have a job to do as a full member of their loved one's care team. You all have jobs to do and yours is to learn all you can about your loved one's situation and act as their advocate.

You are there not only to represent your loved one but also to put a human face to them.

This is a crucial role, for no matter how much they care, your doctor sees at least 25 patients a day, your care manager and therapist have a larger case load than ever and other members of a hospital or care facilities team probably have never even laid eyes on your loved one. Although telemedicine and telehealth are extremely important options these days, personalization through a video screen creates its own challenges.

Over the years, we have found three significant common traits among the caregivers who are being listened to and respected in today's healthcare system. The first is that they must believe that they can make a difference. Secondly, they see their role in their loved one's care as being just as important as any of the professional caregivers. And thirdly, they ask questions. They ask lots of questions. They research and do not easily take "no" for an answer. They become Fearless Caregivers.

A Fearless Caregiver is one who asks questions of their doctor and does not rest until they receive clear and concise answers. A Fearless Caregiver knows their rights concerning their loved one's insurance plan and can exercise those rights. A Fearless Caregiver is one who knows how to find the latest treatment options and present qualified research to the members of his or her loved one's care team. A Fearless Caregiver IS a member of their loved one's care team.

Introduction

I know that so many of you have already become personal advocates for your loved one's care. But, do you know what the very first step to such care is – it is caring for yourself. I can hear you saying as you read these words "who has time to care for me, I spend all my time caring for him (or her)?" My answer to that is, who will step in and care for you AND your loved one when you take ill due to exhaustion or simply not caring for yourself. See, Job One for any caregiver is to make sure that we are taken care of, too.

At a Fearless Caregiver Conference held in Palm Beach County, Florida, that fact came alive for me as well as all caregivers in attendance. The weather that day was as close to being a tropical storm as it could be without the news stations going into full soap-opera interruption mode. I had broken three of my cardinal rules about hosting these events and they are: stay north in the warm months, south in the cold months, and avoid Florida during the hurricane season. Thankfully, there was a lull in the weather during the time that people normally arrive, and we had a packed house of hundreds of caregivers.

As the applause died down after our luncheon speaker's session ended, I took the stage and before I was able to utter a word, heard someone cry from the audience," Is there a doctor in the house?" Not something you want to hear at any event, let alone one you are hosting.

I stopped the proceedings and went to the center of the room to find a nicely dressed gray haired lady slumped over in her chair. There were no doctors in the house but plenty of nurses and as I reached the table, two of them were already assessing the situation. The lady mentioned that she felt like she was going to pass out. We immediately called 911. The lady was at the event with her husband, a gentleman sitting calmly next to her who was living with Alzheimer's disease, and she was, of course, most concerned about his care. The paramedics suggested she go to the hospital with them, but she refused. They insisted, stating that she would probably just relapse once she got home. They had a hard time getting any information from her and finally she told them she had a son who lived in town. He was contacted and advised to meet his parents at the hospital. As she left, she told one of my associates that she stays up all night worrying about her husband and that she never takes care of herself. Some of her friends coaxed her to attend the event knowing that she needed help, but was not willing to accept any and hoped that she could learn something while at the event, about the importance of taking care of herself as a caregiver while at the conference. I think we all did.

We caregivers must certainly learn all we can about the disease or illness that our loved ones are battling, in this case, knowledge truly is power --- but we must also learn all we can about our role as a caregiver – A Fearless Caregiver.

The first act of any Fearless Caregiver is to assess your resources. Is there a sister, brother, neighbor or professional service that can stand in for you a few hours a week or maybe a weekend every few months? Do you know what community services are available to anyone in your situation? Do you even know where to start looking? As an attendee at a Fearless Caregiver Conference stated,

"The cemetery is filled with irreplaceable people."
Who takes over when the irreplaceable caregiver is gone? If you do not believe you have the right to take care of your own needs, you may need a caregiver yourself.

A SOCIETY OF FEARLESS CAREGIVERS

According to Webster's dictionary: the descriptions of the word FEARLESS includes:

1. Calmly resolute in facing dangers or perils
2. Invulnerable to fear or intimidation.
3. Spirited and original…

There is a specific reason that our first book (*The Fearless Caregiver: How to Get the Best Care for Your Loved One and Still Have a Life of Your Own*) and the conferences we host are all entitled Fearless Caregiver. It is because, as a family caregiver, you are the central force for all things that happen for your loved one and should not just become an active member of your loved one's care team but actually be seen as a team leader. For in all intents and purposes, a Fearless Caregiver is also a professional caregiver: as important as the case manager, therapist, nurse or (yes) even doctor.

We have been honored to be able to share the day with family caregivers at nearly 300 Fearless Caregiver Conferences across the nation and look forward to doing so again, soon. As I conjure up the days that I have stood in front of my fellow caregivers at these events, the first thing that comes to mind is the sense of community we are able to create within the four walls of the conference centers. Yet more than that, it is the wisdom shared with one another throughout the day. We all freely share our questions, our fears and even our solutions to the vexing challenges we all face as caregivers. I have heard from so many people that they take the lessons learned out of the conference centers and into the other days during the year.

Just like any other member of our loved one's care team; we need to learn the tools of our trade. What are the first steps to take when you become a new Alzheimer's, Parkinson's, cancer or traumatic brain injury caregiver? What must we know in our second, fifth or even twentieth years of caregiving? What terms and concepts must we learn that will best help our families and ourselves? How do we keep abreast of all the latest and greatest caregiving tools and techniques? How do we keep up to date with the best practices of our professional role as fearless or advocate caregivers? The way to do so is to realize that we are actually the most important piece to the healthcare puzzle for our loved ones and to join up with others who realize that they are also the most important pieces of their own loved ones healthcare puzzle.

We hope the wisdom shared within these pages by your fellow caregivers at the Fearless Caregiver Conferences are of great support as you care for your loved ones. And hopefully care for yourselves as well.

Someday soon, I look forward to spending the day with you at a Fearless Caregiver Conference in your community.

Please stay well, safe and…fearless.

THE FEARLESS CAREGIVER MANIFESTO

Man·i·fes·to (manə ˈfestō)
n. pl. man·i·fes·toes or man·i·fes··tos
A public declaration of principles, policies, or intentions.
intr.v. man·i·fes·toed, man·i·fes·to·ing, man·i·fes·toes
To issue such a declaration.

Your loved one's doctors live by the Hippocratic Oath, the social workers by the Code of Ethics, and the nurses, by the Florence Nightingale pledge. As these other members of the team have codes of ethics and principles to live by as healthcare professionals, we caregivers also need and deserve our own guiding set of principles.

The Fearless Caregiver Manifesto:

- I will fearlessly assess my personal strengths and weaknesses, work diligently to bolster my weaknesses and to graciously recognize my strengths.

- I will fearlessly make my voice be heard with regard to my loved one's care and be a strong ally to those professional caregivers committed to caring for my loved one and a fearless shield against those not committed to caring for my loved one.

- I will fearlessly not sign or approve anything I do not understand and will steadfastly request the information I need until I am satisfied with the explanations.

- I will fearlessly ensure that all the necessary documents are in place in order for my wishes and my loved one's wishes to be met in case of a medical emergency. These will include Durable Medical Powers of Attorney, Wills, Trusts and Living Wills.

- I will fearlessly learn all I can about my loved one's healthcare needs and become an integral member of his or her medical care team.

- I will fearlessly seek out other caregivers or care organizations and join an appropriate support group; I realize that there is strength in numbers and will not isolate myself from those who are also caring for their loved ones.

- I will fearlessly care for my physical and emotional health as well as I care for my loved one's, I will recognize the signs of my own exhaustion and depression, and I will allow myself to take respite breaks and to care for myself on a regular basis.

- I will fearlessly develop a personal support system of friends and family and remember that others also love my loved one and are willing to help if I let them know what they can do to support my caregiving.

- I will fearlessly honor my loved one's wishes, as I know them to be, unless these wishes endanger their health or mine.

- I will fearlessly acknowledge when providing appropriate care for my loved one becomes impossible either because of his or her condition or my own and seek other solutions for my loved one's caregiving needs.

You Are Not Alone: Real World Solutions for Family Caregivers

CARING FOR ONE ANOTHER

I will fearlessly develop a personal support system of friends and family and remember that others also love my loved one and are willing to help if I would let them know what they can do to support my caregiving.

CARING FOR ONE ANOTHER

Go Ask Alice

I was reminded recently of a Fearless Caregiver Conference we held in Los Angeles many years ago. It was a motivating, educating, tearful, happy and spiritual day. Among the awards presented at the event, was one to Ms. Alice Blackman, a family caregiver who still found time to care for others in need in her community. Many tears flowed when Alice's daughter stepped onto the stage to surprise her, having flown down from northern California for the presentation during her lunch break and having to turn around and return to work, later the same day.

I bring Alice to your attention, because in her remarks, she talked about how very important her support group has become to her. At first, she felt forced to go to the support group meeting and sat in the room with her arms crossed and toes tapping, wondering what she was doing, sitting among strangers who seemed to be whining about their lives. How were they ever going to help her as a caregiver? For some reason, Alice went back a second and third time, Lo and behold, after the third session, she was hooked. Alice now says that she doesn't know how she was able to cope before discovering the group and mentioned that the entire group had come to the conference to cheer her on. Alice confirmed once again that we had truly found the right person for the award, due to the fearlessness in which she approaches all she does as a caregiver. She instinctively knew that she needed to find this group and that no matter how uncomfortable she felt during the first two visits, she needed to keep going back.

The only problem Alice's statement presented for me was that I needed to quickly revamp part of the speech which I was to give an hour later, so it wouldn't seem like I was riding on her coattails. It turns out that her support group revelation mirrors almost word for word my comments on the same subject.

Alice is a living example of what I like to call taking a "Leap of Faith." Find an appropriate support group and go three times, no matter what you feel about your first two visits. I guess she is living proof that it works.

Hey, don't take my word for it, Go Ask Alice.

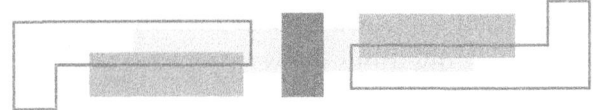

CEO of Caring

I have been talking about family caregivers being the CEO of Caring for My Loved One, Inc. since late last century in Today's Caregiver magazine, on caregiver.com and at the Fearless Caregiver Conferences. Like many CEOs, you have tools at your disposal; but unlike most CEOs, there was no university to go to or MBA to obtain to learn these tools. Your ascendency to the executive level most likely came with a jolting telephone call in the middle of the night telling you that your loved one has just been in an accident, or with the call from the doctor's office to let you know the results of the tests recently taken. That call transports you through the looking glass, where everyone else is talking in jargon that you don't understand and that every decision is potentially of the life and death variety. So, what do you do?

Four Rules of becoming CEO of My Loved One, Inc.

- First: take a deep breath and count to 10. The fact is, with 66.7 million other caregivers in the nation, you are not alone.
- Second: marshal your resources, learn all you can about your loved one's illness or disease – in caregiving, knowledge is truly power.
- Third: find your way to others in your community (or online) who are caring for clients and loved ones.
- Fourth: as any good CEO will tell you, the most important tools you have as a family caregiver are to ask questions of everyone, and to never take a dismissive or an easy no for an answer.

As an example of Rule Number Three:

I refer you to the Fearless Caregiver Conference we held in New Haven, Connecticut many years ago. One of the caregivers in attendance, Stephanie, had been trying to convince her mother that in-home care was needed. The thing that helped is when Stephanie adjusted her attitude to realize that she was (as we say) the CEO of Caring for My Loved One, Inc. and that her mother was her organization's primary client. From then on, things became easier for her when it came to in-home care. Stephanie would hold "client meetings" with her mother and tell her, "You are the lady of the house–it is your house and you are in charge—you are the boss." Each time Stephanie sat down with Mom, the Chairperson of the Board, Mom asked for more things that she would like the in-home caregivers to do for her.

P.S. Stephanie also changed her language to match her mother's history. Before her Alzheimer's diagnosis, her mom had been a bank president and although at first was adamantly against having in-home care, she was quite accepting when Stephanie started referring to the homecare aides as her mom's "administrative assistants".

The reason I bring up Stephanie's story is that, fast-forwarding years into the future and a thousand miles away (at a recent Fearless Caregiver Conference), a male caregiver told me that he had been making himself bald by pulling out his hair trying to get his dad to accept in-home care a few years ago. That was the year he heard me talk about what Stephanie had done- puzzle solved. Baldness prevented. His dad is still happily living at home with in-home care.

CEOs for Caring for Your Loved Ones, Inc., please step up and receive your M.B.A. degree:

Masters of Being AWESOME

There's Snow Place Like Home

On a trip home after a conference in the northeast, I found myself stranded by the (as the media puts it) *BLIZZARD OF THE YEAR*, which, to me, seemed just a tad presumptive, since it is only three weeks into January. My cabin row mates were George and Julie Fox, a middle-aged couple from Pennsylvania, and together we endured a five hour tour of the airport tarmac, with the plane slowly inching towards the de-icing station until the weather became so bad that take-off was no longer an option and we returned to the now-closed airport.

As we took advantage of the waiting time to get to know one another, I was reminded of our regular advice to caregivers, 'Never miss an opportunity to talk with other caregivers in hospital waiting rooms, doctor's offices, pharmacy lines and even on airplanes.' Conversation with the Foxes included George's challenges with getting his dad to stop driving, Julie's taking care of George during and after his stroke six years ago at 42 years of age and long-term care options for Julie's mom.

George told me how he succeeded in guiding his extended family into a unified care team by making sure that each member was tasked with handling specific details which took into consideration their abilities and interests.

When it became clear that we would all be in danger of sleeping at the airport that night, I used my cell phone to find a hotel with rooms in the downtown area while Julie made calls to rebook the three of us for the first flight out on Sunday. To make a long story (and night) short, we developed (with two of their other friends) the camaraderie and teamwork that is possible for strangers to acquire when faced with emergency situations. Together, we all found rooms, shared stories and cell phones and when we returned to South Florida the next morning, after searching in vain for their bags at the airport, I raced them to the port where they managed to catch their ship for a now much deserved cruise.

The only other times that I remember having this kind of quick and constructive bonding with strangers was as a caregiver, waiting through those long nights in the local hospital emergency room. Then as now, we shared stories, caregiving tips and made friendships that have lasted for years. In those cold and uncomfortable hospital waiting rooms, I discovered that in any healthcare situation, the best caregiving expertise is available not only from the people in white coats, but also from your fellow caregiver sitting next to you. And who knows, you may even enjoy the wait.

Surviving the COVID-19 Roller Coaster

When I was a small boy living in South Florida, during the summers we would take trips to visit family members in New York where my mom grew up. I especially loved going to Coney Island. As well as the bright lights, games and (way too much) cotton candy, my favorite thing was to go on the largest wooden roller coaster- The Cyclone.
I remember sitting in the cars which clinked and clanked up to the top of the ride, waiting to plunge down after reaching the top. Then wending our way through hair-raising twists and turns only to be safely deposited at the end of the ride in a disheveled and giggling mess.

When I look at the graphs showing the COVID-19 timelines as it spent the past few months decimating the countries affected before the United States, it brought this roller-coaster ride to mind. As we sat in our cars waiting for our turn up the hill, we watched the cars in line ahead of us with great interest as they went through the hair-raising parts, the slow parts and even as their ride started to slow down at the end.

We in the US, apparently have yet to reach the top of the ride before the plunge. The curve on the graphs seen on television representing the timelines for Italy or China or South Korea all almost exactly overlap, from duration to intensive effects of the virus. These countries started this dreadful ride before us, with all of its stomach-churning twists and turns.

I don't know how long this will take before things are better, or what is about to happen to us in the United States. The only thing I do know is that the way we will get through this successfully is – together.

This year, we are all Fearless Caregivers.

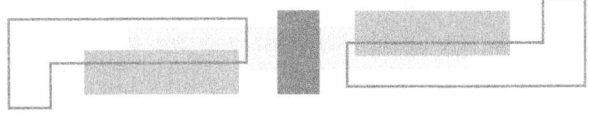

WTMT

So much in our lives have changed over the past few weeks, including the twin and opposing challenges faced by our loved ones dealing with social isolation or too much family time.

With regards to isolation of our senior loved ones, we need to do as much as possible to keep them involved, including Face-timing with the grand-kids and Zoom family gatherings. Remind your senior loved ones that the scammers are out in force now and their bank or insurance company would never ask them for their personal identifiable information like birthday or social security number. They already have it. Tell them to let you know if they are receiving any such calls and generally let any call from an unknown number go to the answering machine. Remember to pay attention to their health and the health of their beloved pets. Reminisce with them. Remind them how much they are loved.

On the flipside, there is also WTMT (Way Too Much Togetherness), as we are sheltering in place with loved ones for who knows how long. This may be the perfect time to take some of those long boiling cups of emotional resentments off the high heat and bring them down to simmer (or at least low heat).

Negotiation, mediation, resolution, love and even counting to ten before speaking, will go a long way to peaceful coexistence, as we are spending WTMT with family members. I'm certainly not naive enough to suggest that we all just forgive and forget old wounds which may surface during these stressful times. Things of this nature are usually a whole lot more complicated than that. We all need to put off that which is not important, such as who said what to whom at the company holiday party. A general rule of thumb should be to avoid those things that are not important to deal with right now including anything not having to do with surviving past this pandemic.

Yet, I contend that, for some people this may be a very good time to calmly, mindfully, honestly and fearlessly discuss some of these long-forgotten wounds to hopefully help them heal, once and for all.

Please remember that your little pitchers not only have big ears, but they also have big eyes. You have the ability to ensure that this time in their lives is filled with either positive or painful memories. So, look over your shoulder and think before you speak. Also, no stress should ever be enough to lead anyone to lay a hand on another in anger. One suggestion to reduce stress in these extraordinary times is to limit the amount of time you watch politicians and pundits on television to the bare minimum. Change the channel, open a book, find a happy song and even dance with your loved ones. Take appropriately socially distanced walks. Exercise at least once a day. Make sure to all laugh together at least once a day. And care for one another.

This year, we are indeed, all Fearless Caregivers.

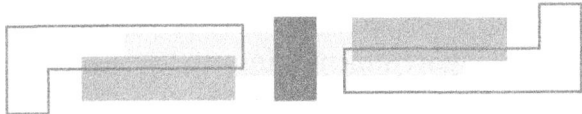

Leading with Love

This year so far, the separation between people who are actively caring for loved ones and those who are not yet doing so, is much less defined than ever.

Now, it is not just family caregivers whose lives have been swiftly upended with no reasonable end in sight. Now, this virus has made all our relationships with loved ones either better or more fragile. Now, we all are regularly thinking of the health and well-being of our loved ones. Now, the strength of our local healthcare system is something that is concerning to all, as it is not when everyone is well. I think this is an important teaching opportunity for family caregivers. We can help our friends, neighbors and family members through the type of fear and uncertainty that we caregivers face daily.

- We can show our friends, neighbors and family members what it means to try and be prepared for any healthcare outcome
- We can help teach our friends, neighbors and family members the importance of interacting with others in times of duress
- We caregivers and carers have long known the value of two sets of three words to get us through the tough times. When talking with your loved ones do not forget to say *I Love You* as often as possible, and when encountering roadblocks when dealing with the system (financial, healthcare, government, insurance) remember the indispensable three words are *Who's Your Supervisor?*

There are so very many things that are shared by all peoples in all nations around the globe: the extraordinarily thin layer of ozone which separates us from the blackness of space, love of our friends and family members, a good laugh, hugs and even the global ecology which we all share. And in regular times, these shared elements of humanity are not usually recognized. There are precious few times that we can see ourselves as all hurtling together in this Spaceship Earth and this is, for better or worse, one of these times.

As any caregiver can tell our friends, neighbors and family in these days in which we find ourselves, the best thing we can do is lead with love.

A Bonus Epiphany

Usually when I travel, I am blessed to be able to meet people who open my eyes to the techniques they employ to help them navigate their caregiving. It may be the six year old girl sitting next to me on the plane with the wisdom of the ages behind her eyes as she tells me all about helping her mommy care for her granny, or the cabbie who has found as many shortcuts to navigating his city's healthcare system as he did for navigating it's streets. But generally, I am only privy to one such lesson per trip, so imagine my surprise, when a bonus lesson popped up.

I received an email from a young man named Ryan who was at a South Dakota conference with his mom. I remembered him from the event. We met in the hall after my speech and talked for a while. He told me how much he enjoyed the event and how much he learned. In his teens and in a wheelchair, his mom never seemed as if she was his caregiver, more like his partner in information gathering. We spoke of how he and his mom never missed an opportunity to gather data at these events regarding his situation. They then go home and pour over the materials to keep themselves abreast of the latest information.

In his email, he told me how he appreciated when I spoke about finding wisdom from the caregivers you meet along the way. He went a step further and told me that he has never had a conversation with anyone where he did not learn something: doctor, fellow conference attendee or ice cream vendor, there was something to learn from everyone who ever crosses your path.

He may not realize this but since his email, I have been trying to follow his words and learn from every single encounter. And you know what? It really works. There is truly a tremendous amount of wisdom in this world and it took me flying across the country to meet Ryan to pay attention.

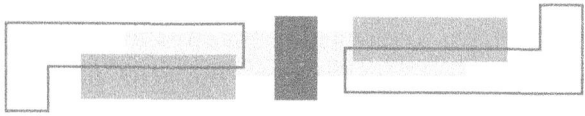

Living Examples

While speaking at family caregiving events, I always ask each member of the audience to take the opportunity to spend time with the experts leading the sessions, as well as the service providers in the room. These professionals have a tremendous amount of experience and wisdom to share and are usually anxious to answer questions. I also tell them to look around the room and remember to talk with the true experts in caregiving among them, their fellow caregivers.

As caregivers, it's vital that we interact with the other care professionals on our loved one's care team, but it is possibly even more important that we take time to interact with one another. What a wasted opportunity it is for us to stand in the pharmacy lines, sit in emergency waiting rooms and even wait for hospital elevators with others who are caring for loved ones and not spend time speaking with them. I guarantee you that in each of these conversations you are going to be surprised at what you will learn to help you as a caregiver and even more surprised at what you will be able to teach your fellow caregiver.

I always learn something when talking with family caregivers. As I was discussing some options to ensure family involvement with our attendees at the Minneapolis Fearless Caregiver conference, one caregiver raised her hand and told us of the monthly potluck dinners she would hold while caring for her mother at home.

All her family members were invited to attend. At first, only four or five would show up, but after a while, people were driving in from neighboring states and some of her parties had over thirty-five family members joining in. Even if caregiving was not a major topic of discussion at each of these soirees, the family members were able to see her mom on a regular basis, which ended much of the misunderstanding starting to occur between herself and her siblings. After hearing her story, a family caregiver sitting in the row ahead of her said that she was sure this was the answer to her own family challenges and that she would host her first family event within the month. Caregivers sharing wisdom with caregivers, now that's the way it should be.

As long as we are still sheltering-in-place, a virtual potluck will also work!

Bette's Brainstorms

I was in Atlanta for a television interview, book signing and to attend a meeting on end-of-life care with the Huntington's Society of America, so I winged into the city pretty sure of my schedule and to whom I would be talking during my short stay.

Well, like everything else I've learned about caregiving, things do not always go exactly as planned and wisdom is found in a wide variety of places and faces. I arrived at the television studio early Monday morning and as I waited in the green room, I met Bette. I'm still not sure what role Bette played at the station, but when we met, she greeted me with an incredibly warm hug, so I think whatever they are paying her, it is not enough.

After my interview, the show producer asked if I would sign a copy of The Fearless Caregiver for Bette. It turns out that not only is Bette taking care of her mother, but she just found out that her daughter was diagnosed with cancer and her favorite nephew was recovering from a serious automobile accident.

Despite all of this, Bette radiated a peaceful and calm presence that was felt by everyone around. As we left the studio, she began to share her story. She said that she visited daily the long-term care facility where her mother lived and spent the rest of the day with her mom.

But Bette was not there to simply sit and visit. As she walked around the facility, she noticed that the soiled sheets were kept on the resident's beds well into the afternoon. When she asked the facility management about this, they said there was only one person changing the beds and it took her all day. Bette had a brainstorm. She suggested that the CNA's who got the residents out of bed could take the sheets off, instead of having the dirty sheets sit on the bed all day. The management's reaction was that they never did it that way before.

They should have known Bette better. Within a week, the system was changed. Bette also noticed that some of the residents who eat more slowly than others were sitting alone while finishing their meals. She quickly put together a schedule of interested families who would sit with these slow eaters until they finished. Bette also set about creating a resident's family council to ensure better communication between families and administration.

Bette's brainstorms have made things appreciably better for the residents at her mother's facility. She is proof of what a motivated caregiver can accomplish.

Once A Caregiver...

We spent a wonderful if not somewhat drizzly day with a room full of newly minted Fearless Caregivers at the Nashville Fearless Caregiver Conference. There were so many lessons learned from the family and professional caregivers we met that I could fill many newsletters with their advice (and probably will).

The first lesson I learned was at dinner the night before with some new friends who came in from Indianapolis to join us for the day. One gentleman was talking about his mother Dora, a retired nurse, who after learning about her neighbor Rose's recent stroke, took it upon herself to design a personalized rehabilitation program and bring it into Rose's bedroom where she was recuperating.

Dora had constructed a story book out a sheaf of lined paper consisting of drawings she had made to illustrate the story of *Jack and Jill*. For many weeks, she sat with her neighbor stroking her paralyzed arm and face and guiding Rose as she both recited and re-wrote out the words to the well-known nursery rhyme.

A few months later when visiting his mother, Rose's daughter took my friend aside and showed him a massive stack of papers where Rose had methodically written and re-written the words to the children's story under the patient tutelage of his mother. By the time he stood there flipping through the pages in disbelief, Rose had recuperated to the point that she showed little sign of the stroke.

The moral of the story: We should never underestimate the healing power of caring, for either the care recipient or the caregiver.

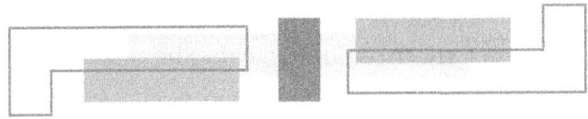

Caregiver Jujitsu

Caregiver Jujitsu - / kair-giv-er ju•jit•su / —a method developed to help caregivers take advantage of important resources by turning their negative responses into positive action.

At a recent Midwest conference, I was pleased to hold an impromptu interview with a caregiver named Susan about one of my favorite subjects, support groups. Susan explained the efforts she made to prompt her brother-in-law, Howard, to go to a local MS spousal support group. Susan's sister had been diagnosed twenty years ago and her condition had worsened steadily over the past five years.

Susan recounted how difficult it was to get Howard to take her suggestion of joining a support group seriously, since he was (in his words) "not interested in sitting around with a bunch of people whining about their painful situations, I've got my own, thanks." As long as the focus of conversation was on how important a support group would be to his own health and well-being, he would have none of it.

Being thoughtful as well as clever, Susan told him about how when she was in a support group for Alzheimer's caregivers a few years ago, she heard advice that the doctors could never have offered. People in the group talked about who were the best practitioners in the area, where free services were offered in the community and tips for what to do when her mom wouldn't eat. She also told him of the interview I held many years ago with Dana Reeve in Today's Caregiver magazine in which Dana told us that some of the best advice she heard as a caregiver came from her own support group.

Susan refrained from talking about how beneficial it would be to Howard's own well-being to join a support group, but emphasized the important things he could learn in a group which would help him become an even better caregiver to his wife. Bingo, he joined the next week. Now, he talks to Susan constantly about his little support group family and how it has saved his life. Hmm, go figure. Caregiver Jujitsu strikes again.

Anger Management

The issue of anger was brought up by an attendee in South Florida which opened a floodgate of feelings and great advice from panel and audience alike. The response from one of our panelists, Laura Zel Kremer, a social worker who is the Caregiver Counselor at MorseLife Health System in West Palm Beach, was, "Of course you are angry, you've saved all your life and were expecting your retirement to be a lot different than it turned out to be when this disease came around…you got a raw deal. You need to accept and understand this and begin to channel your energy to make the best of it for you and your loved ones."

Some of the caregivers had suggestions for how they deal with anger:

- "I walk around the block when I feel that I am going to say or do something I will regret."
- "I will never hesitate to look into my husband's eyes and say I'm sorry when I need to do so."
- "I have my best friend's number on speed dial and punch it rather than the wall."
- "I try to find something to laugh about, preferably with my loved one."
- "I write down my feelings and it makes it easier for me to figure out what I am really angry about"
- "There is something wrong if you don't feel angry at some time during your caregiving. It's what you do about it that makes the difference."

And my personal favorite answer, "Chocolate," which in moderation and medically approved can be just what the doctor ordered.

Break the Glass

I've had many conversations with attendees about what it takes to become a "successful caregiver." This is an important conversation for us to be having in this country at this moment. Talking about what makes a successful family caregiver is focusing on the needs of the caregiver, and that's a good thing, indeed. But, so much of the recent dialog about what makes a caregiver successful concentrates on developing a state of mind that would lead to results sometime in the future, although, this is great, so very little is focused on the here and now. "What can I do to help me get through the day - today?"

So, I began to wonder if we could develop a caregiver's emotional "First Aid Kit," quick and easy things that we caregivers could do to lift our spirits in a pinch. If you find it to be of value, please print it out and put it in a place you will find it when needed. In other words, feel free to "Break the Glass" in times of emergency.

1. **Smile**, it's not funny how often we forget to do this simple act and how well it lifts our spirits
2. **Call someone who makes you feel good**, especially if you haven't spoken with them in a long time
3. **Have a bite of something sinfully delicious**, while being conscious of your own dietary limitations. When was the last time you treated yourself to a snack?

4. **Take a bubble bath,** once you make sure that your loved one is safe and secure, nothing expresses caregiver self-care better than a leisurely bubble bath
5. **Read, pick up that novel or re-read that motivating poem.** When was the last time you turned off the television, turned down the phone and read something nice? (P.S. this tip goes very well with tip number 3)
6. **Buy yourself some flowers.** You deserve it and the sight and smell of something beautiful and fragrant will give you a reason to smile (see number 1)
7. **Take a walk** at a pace that allows you to feel the energy of the wind washing over you
8. **Go online.** You can explore different places, find new friends and learn new things. Make the Internet your getaway when you can't get out of the house

Pinkies Up for Caregivers

Each year in May brings the celebration of National Etiquette Week. I remember the first time I heard about it was after it was already over. I didn't notice any increased etiquette around me that week; but since the week ended on a Friday the 13th, I think people just were trying their best to keep the evil spirits away.

Frankly, I think attention being paid to how we treat one another is a tremendous idea, starting with one week and hopefully lasting throughout the year.

According to the founders of the celebration:
National Etiquette Week is the national recognition of etiquette and protocol in all areas of American life—business, social, dining, travel, technology, wedding and international protocol. The week will raise awareness of all people to act with courtesy, civility, kindness, respect and manners as well as rally people to act with good manners in their everyday lives.

Wonderful sentiment, but may I add one additional area of life—how about etiquette towards family caregivers? It would be wonderful if those around us regularly adhered to some customs of civility towards family caregivers and our loved ones. For example:

- Don't assume that the person in the wheelchair cannot be engaged in your conversation. Remember to make eye contact with the person in the chair as well as the person behind the chair.

This goes double for our loved ones' medical professionals
- We caregivers are not just the person bringing our loved ones to their appointments; we are normally integrally involved with their care and should be treated as equal members of their care team
- If you hesitate to call a family caregiver because you don't know what to say; pick up the phone and try talking about anything but family caregiving; it would be a welcome relief
- If you can't figure out what to do for your friend or loved one who is a family caregiver, make a specific suggestion: "I'm cooking a special meal for you and your family this coming Tuesday." "Hey, I'm going to the drug store. Do you need anything?" These are both good starts

Hmmm…etiquette towards family caregivers? Pass the finger bowl. I think I'm going to like this custom.

Holmes for the Holiday

For caregivers who are looking forward to a holiday visit home to see your caregiving loved ones when such a trip is once again possible, may I be so bold as to offer a few suggestions.

Although it would be a bit inappropriate to walk into your loved one's home with an old trench coat, large magnifying glass in hand and sporting a Sherlock Holmes Deerstalker hat, nevertheless, my dear Watson, you are on a case—the case I call "The Holiday Visit of the Caregiver Detective." (Cue organ crescendo.)

When there, you need to be inquisitive without becoming an inquisitor, but you might want to take some time to look around the home for safety issues including the following:

Stairs
- Is there damaged or loose carpet on the stairway?
- Is the stairway well lit?
- Are there any loose banisters?
- Is there any way to rearrange the home setting to reduce or even cancel the need for your loved one to walk upstairs?

Bathrooms
Most emergency room visits from senior citizens occur due to falls in the bathroom.
- Peek into the medicine cabinets and refrigerator for old medicines or foods.
- Are there throw rugs on the floor without proper backing?

- Are there grab rails where needed? (A towel rack will do no good in a fall.)
- Is there proper seating in the shower?

Hold Caregiver Board of Director meetings with your fellow family members who will also be visiting.

Create a holiday care plan for your caregiving loved one so he or she can get out of the house to take some time for themselves while you are there.

If your loved one lives in a rural area:

Isolation
Although a psychological challenge for many urban caregivers, isolation is also a physical challenge for many rural caregivers since they possibly live far from others.

Check to see if they are becoming too isolated.
How often do they?
- See friends,
- Go to church,
- Go to doctor visits, etc.

Are there any transportation services available to them?

Home Modification
Homes that were perfect for raising children now can become hazardous for seniors to get around.

Find out about local services for home modification to safeguard them in their home.

Be sure your loved one understands that your goal is the same as theirs—to make the home as safe as can be, so they can live there as long as possible.

Safety
The work it takes to maintain a farm can become too dangerous for seniors.

Spend time with your senior loved one as they do their chores, to assess for difficulties and dangers.

Before you visit
Discover what local service organizations serve your loved one's community and reach out to these organizations yourself.

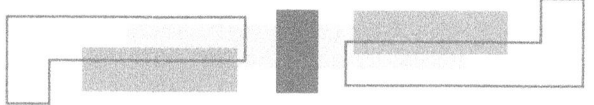

Celebrity Caregiver Wisdom

DANA REEVE

Gary Barg: How do you deal with stress?

Dana Reeve: Stress is an ongoing problem. I find Yoga is really helpful, but then I find my life gets so stressed out, that I don't have time for Yoga. No time for the cure. It's ironic, one of the things I speak on is nurturing the nurturer. I really believe in it. I was telling a friend of mine that I was going to speak on it, and she looked at me and said, "Better start practicing what you preach." I do think you can deal with stress in little ways, you can give yourself little getaways, and it doesn't always have to cost money. It's really a gift you have to give yourself: mini respites.

Gary Barg: What do you do for your "mini respites"?

Dana Reeve: Yoga is great when I take the time. But even when I don't, I would just go up into a room where no one will come in and do whatever it takes, whether it's reading, sitting completely quietly or doing something where I'm not reporting to someone: not answering the phone, not getting something for someone, just locking myself away. Taking a bubble bath, even a mental bubble bath.

Gary Barg: What's been your best source of reliable information as a caregiver?

Dana Reeve: Other caregivers. Over the past few years, I've talked to a lot of women whose husbands are injured, sharing tips and ideas, and venting with one another. You get advice from your doctors, or you get the official recommended procedure on some things, and then someone else will come in and say, "Oh, you know what's easier?" Or they'd say, "Well yes, you can spend all this money on this particular kind of bandage, or you can cut up a Maxi pad, and it sticks to the sock." I get all of this useful information about so many different products that are helpful. Everything from machines to suppositories.

Gary Barg: Chris mentioned in Still Me, that only 30% of people will fight their insurance company, Do you have any advice for the rest?

Dana Reeve: Yes. My first piece of advice is, "Don't take it personally." When I first started fighting the insurance company, I used to scream and cry, "How can they be doing this to us?" Then I realized they do it to everybody. My second piece of advice is, when people ask, "Can I do anything to help?", assign them writing letters to the insurance companies after you get denials. Writing re-submissions becomes an incredibly valuable thing that someone can do for you. It's amazing how much it will ease your mind. Whenever someone asks if they can help me, I ask them to do something specific, and it gets done. I think that people want to help, even busy people.

Gary Barg: What positive things do you see in motion for caregivers?

Dana Reeve: As caregivers we're working primarily out of a feeling of love and obligation toward the person for whom we care. But that's also when we become invisible. We don't see it as a job, it's just part of our life. But it is a job and there should be tax breaks, as well as other kinds of assistance. Also, the amount of money family caregivers are saving the healthcare system is tremendous. It's phenomenal, and this is something I don't think people realize. We have to speak out and be counted in a census.

I love this quotation from Rosalynn Carter's book. "There are only four kinds of people in the world: those who have been caregivers; those who are currently caregivers; those who will be caregivers; those who will need caregivers." Truer words have never been spoken.

PHYLICIA RASHAD

Gary Barg: If you only had one piece of advice for somebody about their own healthcare or about caring for their loved one, what would that advice be?

Phylicia Rashad: You must take care of yourself. It is an act of love. You should take care of yourself so that you are really nurturing yourself to have the best to give to others. From my own experience, it is important to take care of one's own self. Not as self-defense, not as an act of revenge or rage, but because it is the right thing to do. If there is no water in the well, you cannot share it with people. If there is no food in the refrigerator, you cannot feed people. If there is no energy in your body, if your mind is in a state of constant distraction or dismay, you cannot be of service to people. And you are not going to be the best company either.

WENDIE MALICK

Gary Barg: You talk about humor and, obviously, you are a great comedic actor; that is part of your makeup. But, I also believe in the value of humor in family caregiving.

Wendie Malick: There is humor in the chemo room, I am telling you. That is what gets people through; it really truly is. I remember when my grandmother, who was just one of the coolest women I ever knew, had to go into an assisted living facility towards the end. At one point, she was on some sort of medication that made her hallucinate and she thought that she was on the Orient Express, traveling around to all of these fabulous cities. My mother said, "Oh, Mom, you were not really there; that was just your medication." She said, "Really? I am hallucinating?" So the next time my mother went to visit her, she asked, "Mom, how is everything going?" My grandmother said "Well, I was going to the dining room and all those people were saying, 'Hello, Helen. How are you Helen? Good to see you.' I just ignored them because I figured they probably were not there anyway."

SCOTT FOLEY

Gary Barg: Scott, if you had to just tell me the one single most important piece of advice you'd like to share with family caregivers, what would that be?

Scott Foley: Man, the one single most important piece of advice I would share with family caregivers would be to remember that you're all in this together. It's so easy to focus on the sick person. That's where all our energy goes. It's great. It should, but you've got to remember that a disease like recurrent ovarian cancer hits not just the sick person. It can take down a family. You've got to take care of yourselves. You have to open your eyes, and don't just look at the sick person, but look to the people around you. Help them and make sure that they are getting everything they need for everyone around them. That's as important as making sure the room is quiet and the person is fed, and they are taking their medication. It is equally as important.

DAN GASBY

Gary Barg: I'd say the most important person in the life of somebody living with a disease or illness is the family caregiver. So I really appreciate you sharing your time with us.

Dan Gasby: When you become a caregiver, it's like when someone loses their sight and the other senses become heightened. When you have to care for someone else, you suddenly understand how important it is to get outside of yourself and see others through different lenses because it's necessary to understand what they're experiencing from the perspective of a third person. And I think that's how wisdom is developed and put into effect.

Gary Barg: You develop a depth of vision that others who haven't been caregivers don't have. There are few things in the world that change you as a human being at the genetic level but I think caregiving's one of those things.

Dan Gasby: You know what? I agree and I think that it heightens everything – the good becomes so much sweeter. And the things that are difficult, you ameliorate them. Not that you can make them go away but you can understand them better and sort of dissect them so that they're not as debilitating to you as the caregiver. I think the most important thing is that you learn how to live in the now.

GETTING HELP FROM OUR LOVED ONES

I will fearlessly honor my loved one's wishes, as I know them to be, unless these wishes endanger their health or mine.

GETTING HELP FROM OUR LOVED ONES

Wish Fulfillment

I am always honored when asked to speak at the annual South Florida Scleroderma conference. As with most of the conferences I have attended, the participants at this event deal with multiple care issues; caring for spouses and children with scleroderma, parents with Alzheimer's, diabetes and strokes and of course, handling their own care issues at the same time. A true "Club Sandwich Generation" crowd.

One year when the conversation came around to the subject of Living Wills. I was particularly taken with a caregiver who raised her hand and said that although she is in favor of Advanced Directives, her wish was to not fill out a DNR (Do Not Resuscitate) form and that all measures were to be taken no matter what medical condition she was in at the time. I had to stop and think about it for a moment, but she was right.

So much of the conversation on advanced directives I have heard over the past few years has to do with a loved one's decision to have a say in the conversation when "enough is enough." But, if the family has had open and honest conversations about a loved one's wishes (or your wishes, for that matter) and a decision has been reached, then whatever the choice, it should be respected and adhered to when the situation arises. If that preference goes against the grain of the rest of the family, so be it. If your loved one was legally able to make the decision regarding his or her end of life care, and if all parties have been heard before the paperwork had been signed, then exercising their wishes at the appropriate time is truly where you can show your love by allowing them to have their voice heard at a time they need it most.

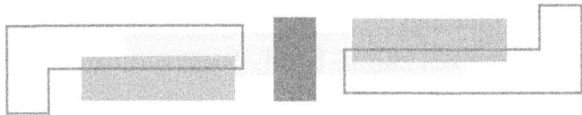

Norma's Nuggets

It was a banner week for me in that I got to do my favorite thing twice. I spoke in Orlando at the World Congress on Disabilities one day and the next, at the Fearless Caregiver Forum in Columbus, Ohio. If you were thinking that there would be great differences in these two audiences, one being at a primarily pediatric disability event and the other with more senior caregivers, you couldn't be more wrong. The juxtaposition of events in such a short period of time just reinforces my feeling that caregivers have much to learn from one another regardless of the disease or illness they are battling.

Some tidbits I picked up:

- In order to share her life with her long-distance friends and relatives, one caregiver sends out regular email messages about some of the lighter moments she can share regarding her mother who is living with early stage Alzheimer's. She calls these missives "Norma's Nuggets"

- One of the participants keeps a journal and saves a special section for letters to those who have been particularly annoying to her that week. After writing the letters, she burns them.
- One attendee told of her arguments with her loved one's doctors, that is, until she started to write down everything the doctor told her, as the doctor was talking. Kind of keeps the docs on their toes.

Every time I talk with caregivers, I get to take home nuggets of gold.

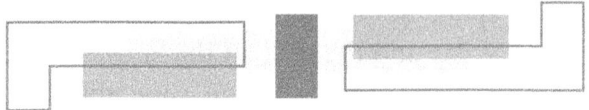

The Driving Issue

I always ask the attendees to hold the driving questions to the last half hour of the event, since it generally swamps all other concerns. My contention is that most families know that their loved one should not be driving for at least six months before acting and their loved ones know they should not be driving for at least a year.

So many times, the challenges include being able to communicate your concerns without your loved one immediately shutting you down, as well as having a viable replacement to the mobility that the car offers. Yet, if you make a list of all the costs associated with driving, including maintenance, fuel, tires, repairs and taxes, you would find that figure represents a significant pool of money that can be applied to solving the transportation challenge. Not to mention the risk associated with having a loved one on the road who shouldn't be wheeling around a ton of metal. One of the concerns that face us as family caregivers is how to take away the keys, hopefully without taking the direct blame for the loss of their car.

We have heard some ingenious methods that caregivers employ when faced with the driving issue, among them:

- Find out what the laws in your state allow in these instances, sometimes you can make an anonymous call and the driver's bureau will call your loved one in for retesting.
- Enlist your loved one's doctor and/or the local police department. This news is always better coming from the professionals.
- Give them a set of non-working car keys and always offer to drive.
- Detach the distributor cap to their car (but remember to let the mechanic in on your scheme).
- Once agreement is made about driving, put a large note in the windshield reminding your loved one that they agreed not to drive.
- Sell their car, although people at more than one event have reported that their loved one simply bought a new one.
- If you talk with your loved one with other family members in the room, rehearse what is to be said. It is much better when everyone is on the same page.

- Create a transportation plan once they can no longer drive, using local services and relatives.
- Remember to put yourself in your loved one's shoes when the time comes to take away the keys. His or her driver's license was a key to independence they received in their youth. We must recognize their fear that taking away the car keys feels like the beginning of the end to them. How would you feel?
- Many times, people know when they can no longer drive; they are just looking for a way to keep their dignity when they give up their license.
- If you are thinking it is time to finally have that talk with your loved one, do it as soon as possible. You probably should have had it six months ago.

Remember it could be worse, one caregiver told us that she was relieved that her 92-year-old father just had his license revoked by the state – his pilot's license.

DRIVING RESPONSES FROM FAMILY CAREGIVERS

Driving

Since we recently moved to Virginia, my husband (who has vascular dementia) would always drive. He cannot drive anymore, and he says he doesn't know where we are going so, I better drive rather than my telling him "turn left or right." So far, it's working.

Loving white lies

Great suggestion from Dayna Thompson at the Alzheimer's Resource Service to a family caregiver who shared the following story about her mother. "I was at a total loss of how to get my mother back home when she left the house to walk to the subway stop and return to her childhood home. I knew better than deny her reality, but I didn't know what else to do. 'Ma., This is Bloomington, Indiana not Budapest, there is no subway!' did not work. No surprise. I only got her to turn back when she got cold."

Dayna suggested that if it happens again, the caregiver should tell her mother, "the subway isn't running today." Brilliant!

Taking the keys

"I had to take the keys from my dad. Hardest thing I have ever done. Had my car parked behind dad's car. As he sat in the driver's seat of his car, I told him that mom was making lunch. (It was 9 a.m.) 'You know how mad mom gets when you're late for eating.' He never wanted mom upset. Took a good 15 minutes to get him out of the car, but the keys "disappeared" after that. I cried all the way home."

One year at the Nashville Fearless Caregiver Conference, a young man stood up and told the attendees how concerned he was about his mom's driving. He did not know how to successfully broach the subject, since, as he said, "she's a very strong lady."

By the time the Area Agency on Aging professional and the elder attorney on the panel were able to respond, at least 10 caregivers offered their clever solutions to their own driving issues, including some listed in this article and a few others such as sitting in the driver's seat whenever a loved one wanted to drive, selling the car and telling them every time they asked that it was in the shop, giving a loved one a set of keys that do not work.

We are thankful that this interaction was videotaped and can be found at the Fearless Caregiver channel on YouTube.

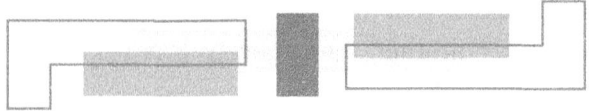

The Couch Conversations

My dad had his own special place on the couch in our living room as I was growing up. Nothing too "Archie Bunker's chair" about this situation. Just anytime the family was sitting on the couch, that was where he sat. And if you were sitting in that space at any other time, it was still known as "Dad's space."

Sometimes late into the night, I used to sit on the other end of the couch talking with him about many varied topics—what happened during the day that was keeping Dad up so late, politics, music, even some of the latest jokes he heard from the guys at his plant. What we never really spoke of was his own childhood. He was born in 1929, spent his early years in Philadelphia and then moved north to the Delaware Valley area of Pennsylvania. He joined the Marines during the Korean War and was stationed in Miami, Florida, when he met my mom.

The living room in question was in North Miami Beach, Florida where I grew up in the 60s and 70s, until moving off for college.

The reason I bring up these couch conversations is that, whenever I would return home to visit after his diagnosis with multiple myeloma in 1990, we resumed these conversations as if no time had passed. One night as I was walking through the living room, I saw him deep in thought. Upon noticing me, he waved me over to sit and started to tell me what he was thinking about.

For the first time, he spoke of his childhood to me. A therapist he had been seeing asked him to think back to the first place he could remember where he felt safe and at peace. She asked him to think back to that place whenever the pain was too much to bear.

Now, Dad was no fan of therapy. In fact, this was the third psychologist he had begrudgingly agreed to see after deciding that the sessions with the previous therapists were a waste of time and that none of them understood him at all. This therapist, however, seemed to hit the spot with this specific exercise.

Dad told me that whenever things would get too stressful as a kid, he would retreat into the woods around his house into a hidden area just the right size to hold a kid and his dreams. There was nothing physically unique about the location—just some sheltering trees and soft grass on a rolling hill—but that was his spot. He smiled as he told me of the time he spent in his own secluded hideout. Although I know that development and the passing decades have erased this private sanctuary, whenever I am in that neck of the woods, I look off into whatever woods I see and wonder...

As we are all sheltering in place with our loved ones – please take the time to have these talks with each other. It may be one blessing to come from these days, as I am still learning so much from my dad's couch conversations.

Keep your Machete Sharp

Gramp was an outstanding artist. My mom, siblings and I have many of his paintings hanging in our homes, including one of a thatched hut village in the Philippines where he was stationed in World War Two. The picture of the village was painted onto a bamboo sifter that the villagers used to clean their rice.

As well as an artist, Gramp was also a craftsman and he firmly believed in using the right tool for the right job. His old wooden tool kit was a world of wonder for his grandchildren to investigate. I was reminded of Gramps toolkit at the 21st annual Fort Lauderdale Fearless Caregiver Conference for a few reasons.

Firstly, we were blessed to be joined by a handful of our 2019 Today's Caregiver Friendly Award winners and I was pleased to present them their awards during lunch. What these folks and every other award nominee and winner over the past 18 years have in common is that they spend their days striving to create better and more efficient tools for family caregivers. Whether it is an animatronic pet developed to help calm our loved ones living with cognitive challenges or an amazing new supportive caregiving book or even a documentary connecting us to the lives of a family as they battle the dreaded Alzheimer's disease, these are now tools that caregivers can have in their own personal toolkits.

Yet, another thing that brought Gramps toolkit to mind, was a phrase (that I've never heard before) shared by our friend Kim Miller of SeniorBridge as she served as an expert Q and

A panelist. Her words were (paraphrasing) "as caregivers we all need to take the time for ourselves to make sure we keep our machetes sharp."

Amen to that!

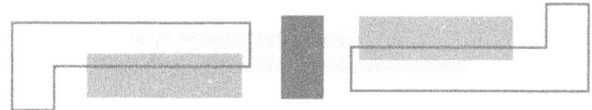

Fearless at Fourteen

The 110th Fearless Caregiver Conference started out of the gate at full gallop. One of the first questions set the tone for the day. A 30-something-year-old goateed man stood up and said, "I'm from up north and my question is about long-distance caregiving. I have a 90-year-old mother who lives here in Boca Raton. I am her only son, yet she is quick to say "Don't bother me" if I offer help. She doesn't believe in doctors. Fiercely independent, she just got her driver's license renewed for five more years. Yesterday, I opened her refrigerator—one can of nuts and four eggs. She is extremely sharp and makes it a point to tell me often. She fell and fractured her pelvis a few years ago, but says it never happened. My issue is that she wants to live independently, but every time I see her, she gets weaker and thinner…I don't know what to do. One of the reasons I came down here at this point is to get some advice from this conference. What can I do?"

Well, I can shamelessly admit that I wait all morning for such a challenge. When a question like this shows up, I like to start what I refer to as "A Caregiver Answer Thread." Instead of going on to the next question after a few answers, we stay on the topic for a while. I certainly got more than I bargained for in responses.

From the expert panelists to the caregivers in the audience, the answers ranged from contacting geriatric care managers, the Area Agency on Aging Elder Help Line and local support groups, to utilizing what I like to call *Caregiver Jujitsu* to try and get her to see that any help is more for your well-being than for hers. And even try to get her to see that she is the CEO of her own care.

But my favorite response came when a hand shot up attached to a most unexpected respondent—a 14-year-old girl. A grandparent caregiver in attendance brought one of her young charges with her and this fresh-faced young lady was ready with some sage advice: "I know I'm really young to know about this, but I think your mom is trying to make you come toward her more rather than push you away. The more trouble she presents to you, the more she would see you in town. I think you need to try hard to see the situation through her eyes."

I presented this teen-sager with a much-deserved button proclaiming "I am a Fearless Caregiver – Don't Mess with Me" which she wore proudly the rest of the day.

If this young lady is any indication of what the next generation has to offer, I think we are all in good, smart, capable and caring hands.

The Beck-and-Call-Giver

I was in Boise, Idaho to keynote a caregiving conference hosted by Friends in Action, a small but energetic organization headed by Stephanie Bender-Kitz, Ph.D. As we always find on the Fearless Caregiver tour each year, being in a large room with your fellow caregivers can be an eye-opening experience—especially when you thought you were the only one going through caregiving in your community.

Once again, I learned as much from the attendees as I did from the expert panel and I truly believe that the panelists will confirm my contention. During the morning Q and A session, a caregiver who had been patiently waiting to talk finally got her chance. She said, "I don't have a question about being a caregiver for my dad; I have a question about being a beck-and-call-giver for my dad."

That got a lot of laughs, but it did ring a bell with some of the caregivers. It seems as if she had a situation where her dad had simply given up and now expects people to be at his beck and call, doing things for him that he could do for himself but had simply decided not to. She has developed a strategy that allows him to do more things, such as making his own sandwiches by simply not being available at lunch or not putting his clothes away so he would have to do it himself.

By carefully allowing him to take on responsibilities appropriate to his abilities, she has given herself some more freedom and has made him feel a tad bit more independent as well.

Three More Little Words

At a recent Fearless Caregiver Conference, I heard from a caregiver who was slapped in the face with the thoughtless comment from several of his relatives that once appropriate facility placement was made for their mutual loved one, he was no longer her caregiver. Whenever I hear this comment, I find that there is only one appropriate three- word response. So here goes…Nonsense, poppycock and baloney! (Please forgive me for such profanity.)

Not only are you still your loved one's caregiver after long term care placement, but you may have added years and quality to their lives as well as saving your own. The other thing you have accomplished is to add members to your loved one's care team.

As far as I am concerned, you are still the captain of that team, responsible for seeing that your loved one receives the best care possible from the facility. But the value you have added to your loved one's well-being by your carefully determined decision has been multiplied. Just consider the realization that it sure would be nice to be able to spend some pleasant time with your loved one as loving son, daughter, husband or wife again.

Now, all family caregivers can be armed with those three little words to respond to those who would utter such unfeeling and thoughtless opinions: Nonsense, poppycock and baloney. Then just turn and walk away.

The Reverse Gift List

If you find yourself in front of an audience of family caregivers and want to get a sure laugh, tell them that you know for a fact that their extended family members are doing all that they can to help them as they care for their loved ones. It is not funny, but so many times, caregiving is a tremendously isolating life event. Yet it doesn't always have to be so.

People do want to help, but we caregivers don't know how to ask them for it / are too ashamed to think that we need anyone's help and don't even know what kind of help to request. In response, we've developed a tool to help caregivers create an informal support team from the people around them in their daily lives.

It is called a *Reverse Gift List,* and the process is quite simple and can be accomplished quite easily: First a caregiver makes two columns on a fresh piece of paper (or computer screen). The first column is entitled "People I trust," and title the second column "Things they can do." In the "People" column, list all the people who you think would do any little thing for you. In the "Things" column, make a list of simple tasks that would help you and your loved one and that frankly you would do for anyone who asked you for the same favor. Then match up the task to person. Allow me to show you an example.

For me it might be:
People: Steven (brother), Nancy (friend), Alie (niece), Phyllis (neighbor), Sally (co-worker).

List of things people can do: Cook dinner for us once a month. Whenever you go to the grocery store, call and see if we might need something, same thing with the pharmacy or cleaners. Have the grandkids call dad each weekend, just to talk. Make calls to the insurance company.

This last one I learned from Dana Reeve conducting a cover interview with her for *Today's Caregiver* magazine. She said that after her husband's accident, they were swamped with insurance challenges that kept her on the phone all day, so when people would ask, "Dana, Can I do anything to help?," she would assign them writing letters to the insurance companies after they got denials. In her own words: "Writing re-submissions becomes an incredibly valuable thing that someone can do for you. It's amazing how much it will ease your mind. Whenever someone asks if they can help me, I ask them to do something specific, and it gets done. I think that people want to help, even busy people."

So, when people ask what they can do to help (or especially if they don't) caregivers can be ready with bite-sized, manageable tasks that will help them and actually make their friends feel good for being able to be of some help. And, having someone watch a caregiver loved one for a few hours while they luxuriate in a long, hot bubble bath counts, too.

It is all there for the asking; we just must change the way we think.

So how do we change the way we think? It's like the old joke: A tourist stops a native New Yorker on the streets of New York and asks, "How do you get to Carnegie Hall?" The answer: "Practice, Practice, Practice.

Sneaky Loving Bits

As we travel the nation talking with our fellow family caregivers, our hope is to help bring the best answers, support and advice to light. We talk about such things as the importance of being able to communicate with our loved ones for whom we care. This is extremely important as we all work so very hard to ensure they eat well, stop driving (if necessary) and even take their medicines as directed.

This effort takes diligence, fortitude and most of all, quite a bit of sneakiness. You heard me correctly, in this case you have my full permission to extend your usual decent and truthful personality to include a bit of, as we say in the old country, Blarney and maybe even a little white lie or two. All in the service of the greater good. In some cases, this is the only way you will be able to do all you can do to keep your loved one safe and secure.

To further extoll the virtue of loving sneakiness as you care for your loved ones, I offer the following suggestions that we have heard from family caregivers over the years. Don't worry, you will have a chance to add your own successful little white lies to the list at the end of this article.

Some Lovingly Sneaky Bits

- When the conversation turned to taking away a loved one's keys during a q and a session, a slight elderly lady raised her hand. She told us in a surprisingly booming voice that if you took the car key to the dealer, they can make a duplicate key which will turn when placed in the ignition, but will not engage the motor. Her husband would go out to the garage for an extended period of time trying to get the car started with this dummy key, and finally come inside asking her to drive him. He was too embarrassed to tell her that he could not start the car.

And from another caregiver:

- After taking care of my husband for several years, it became necessary to put him in assisted living. I visit him five times a week. When I leave, I always do so when it is his lunch or dinner time. That makes my leaving easier on both of us. Also, when I leave, I say I am going to the dentist or getting my hair cut. As he has Alzheimer's, he does not remember that I said it the day before. Sneaky but helpful.

And one from my own experiences

- My grandfather fought the idea of spending time at an adult day care facility until we told him that they hired him to teach art to the other members. As a former art teacher, he was thrilled to go every single day from then on. Sneaky but effective.

Finding Your Tribe

They say ole' dogs don't learn new tricks. Which may certainly be true, but I did learn a new and extremely effective phrase when helping caregivers understand the benefit of joining a support group.

Before the Fearless Caregiver Conference in Evansville, Indiana, I used to talk to caregivers who were worried about joining a support group because they didn't want to sit around and "hear whining about other attendee's caregiving situations" and tell them to go three times to an appropriate and well-led group when you found one.

The first time you go, it very well may seem like you parachuted into a raucous holiday get together of a family you have never met before. The second time, you might start recognizing yourself in the words of your fellow attendees, but I have never heard of a caregiver going to such a group three times and not coming home and jumping on the phone to tell everyone about this wonderful new concept they discovered.

Anyway, it was a very lively, sharing and warm group that cold day (ok, I'm a weather wimp, 50 degrees is cold to me). I was also glad that PASATS, an incredible Parkinson's support organization in the tri-state area was represented. One of their family members stood to answer why support groups are so very important for caregivers and she said in three short words what it takes me at least 10,000 to say. She said that finding the right support group is like "Finding Your Tribe." Boom. Drop the Mic. Walk Away.

We have all known that found tribe feeling before, in school, at church and even with family members. A good support group is a safe and comforting, honest and open place filled with wisdom, advice, shoulders to cry on and even laughter.

Now who wouldn't want to belong to a tribe like that?

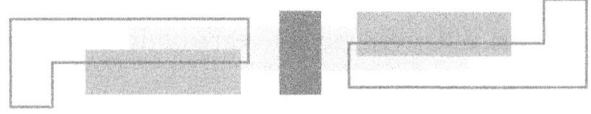

Let's Do the Time Shift Again

At the special Halloween Fearless Caregiver Conference, we held in Port Saint Lucie (our 120th event), the only scary thing was how much wisdom and advice was shared by the family caregivers in attendance. And that's a good scary.

We spoke a lot about one of the most important things you need to have in your caregiver toolkit: how to navigate the holiday season as a family caregiver. This is a topic near and dear to my heart and about which I've been talking to caregivers for many years. Each time I have this conversation, I learn even more from the caregivers in the room. For instance, at this event, we spoke of creating new traditions after a loved one takes ill or even after they pass.

Maybe Dad used to put up all those magnificent decorations, but how about enlisting friends and family members to do so? Make a party out of it. Or Mom (the primary caregiver) always had the family holiday dinner at her house and would not think of altering those plans. Okay, you can keep the intent of her wishes intact, but how about potluck this year with everyone bringing their favorite dishes? And don't forget to solicit help to set up before and clean up after the event.

As Covid-19 is making travel too great a challenge this year, how about time shifting? One gentleman caregiver spoke of how he was able to create last year's holiday event for his wife later in the year and was able to get her two sisters to fly in for the celebration. In fact, one attendee spoke of having multiple birthday dinners for her mother who just turned 95 years old. It was fun for her mom, who asked each time, "Whose birthday are we celebrating?"

One caregiver wanted to visit with her 92-year-old mother in Canada for what could be their last holiday together, but could not figure how to tell her husband (who is living with Alzheimer's disease and for whom the trip would be too great a challenge) that he would not be able to go with her. After she received a lot of help and advice from her fellow caregivers, she said, "I think I always knew how to make this happen but was too wracked with guilt to think it through."

Guilt. Now that's one gift that caregivers don't need, don't deserve and is worthy of being returned as soon as it is delivered.

For the Sake of Mary

On a recent cross-country flight, I sat next to a doctor who was returning from his niece's funeral.

He told me he had been worried about his sister's mental health even before her daughter had taken ill. Mary always picked him up at the airport when he would visit, but in recent years she had stopped because she was losing her way in the city where she had lived her entire life. Her family was concerned, but no one knew what steps to take.

Mary's city is home to a leading memory disorder center, and I told him to make sure she went for a neurological evaluation as soon as possible. The family was interested in helping Mary, but even with all of the health care professionals among them, they were still paralyzed about what steps to take and in what order to take them.

I told him the family's actions would be similar to a physician's medical plan: Diagnose, Assess and Prescribe. First, the diagnosis was made (there was something amiss); then the assessment of what steps to take (What are the available diagnostic options and community resources?); and finally, the prescription (How do you help your loved one realize that an assessment is made not to impede independence, but to be able to retain as much as possible? What are the family plans if the results show signs of a cognitive disorder?).

Most important is to put a timeline to these steps. The family had been discussing her possible memory challenges for at least four years. Our conversation must have crystallized things for him, because he said the family would spend this coming weekend putting a plan in place.

If they do, I can guarantee that this is done for the sake of the entire family and not only for Mary.

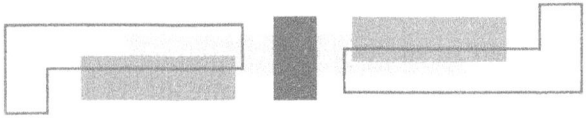

Those Four Little Words

As far as I am concerned, there are two sets of three little words that every family caregiver needs to have at their disposal and use as frequently as possible.

The first set is obvious to you romantics out there—it is, of course, *"I Love You."*

You can't say that enough. Add in a smile and a warm hug for good measure.

Any longtime newsletter reader will already know what the second set of words is and that it must be used unfailingly and fearlessly whenever necessary: *"Who's your supervisor?"*

Those words will work wonders when you face any unreasonable roadblock as you care for your loved one.

At a recent Fearless Caregiver Conference, a family caregiver expanded my caregiving vocabulary. It turns out that she was getting extremely frustrated by having to answer the same questions over and over again from her mother who was living with Alzheimer's disease.

After one such session, she was about to respond angrily to her mom, who would not understand anything but the anger in her daughter's voice. Before she had a chance to speak, her husband (a wise man, indeed) took her aside and said the following four words.

These became the mantra of the event that day. I would like you to say them to yourself whenever those unimportant things that happen make us lose our perspective.

The phrase is: ***"What Does It Matter?"***

Indeed.

Celebrity Caregiver Wisdom

DIXIE CARTER

Gary Barg: What would you say is the most important piece of advice you'd like to share with family caregivers?

Dixie Carter: Caregiving will be unlike anything you will do in your whole life; it's a different endeavor from any other endeavor in life. You, the person doing it, get something very rich; a great, great learning experience. My advice would be trying; say your prayers and try and believe that there will be a response to your needs. Believe that as unlikely as it may seem to you, there will be a response to your need; don't be afraid to ask for it … try.

CARRIE ANN INABA

Gary Barg: We always say that caring for yourself is job one, because who is going to step in and care for you and them when you fall apart because you took yourself out of the circle of care and you are not caring for yourself at all?

Carrie Ann Inaba: Absolutely. It is job one, yes. You have to take care of yourself because without you, if you are the caregiver, what does anybody have? I do believe that the next role is then to help them make good decisions about how they want to take care of themselves and their future, what medical treatments they want to take, what course of action they want to do, and what supplementary health care and alternative therapies are interesting or not interesting. It was actually a very beautiful experience because, as every caregiver knows, there is a bond that reforms, especially when it is your parents. I had not been that close to my parents in a while. By being their caregiver, there are a lot of beautiful moments that happen because you are spending such quality time with someone you care about. I found that to be such a beautiful catalyst, that my mom had cancer. It was such a scary word, but at the same time, so many beautiful things happened. Now my mom is in remission and she is living a healthier lifestyle than she did before she had cancer. She is much more aware of her health, and she has more gratitude towards her health. I guess her overall awareness of health has changed, and I am grateful for that because it makes me feel more confident in the choices she is making in her life and how she is taking care of herself.

RICHARD LUI

Gary Barg: You have four siblings. How did you create a family caregiving plan that works for all of you?

Richard Lui: As you know Gary, siblings don't always get along but for the most part we do get along and I think it just all fell into place. We started a couple of Google docs, one for scheduling and one for what we were learning, so that we wouldn't have to get on conference calls. We were getting on conference calls about once a month early on, and now it's just second nature. But, I think that was key in that we were each volunteering what we could do. And that was the first thing. Each of us, on our first bunch of calls was describing what our limits are, what we could handle, some more, some less. And then we just divided it and tried to battle this. Now it is still very straightforward. It's I can be home this week, not next week. I pick those two to three weeks out of the month that I can be there, then my sister will select those two or three weeks that she can be there. My two brothers who live in the city, would then determine what days they could fit in. So now it's kind of second nature, but earlier on it was very specific. What can you do, what can't you do.

Gary Barg: Well, and by the time it becomes second nature, that's when you really need the support. Anything that they can offer. We call it the Reverse Gift List. Any gift that you can give to caring is valuable. We just have to figure out what pieces we need.

Richard Lui: Right. The difficult part sometimes is saying, well, what you can just do or give, is that enough? I think your statement about everything counts, is the graceful way to look at it. It's tough for every family, I think, when you're going through that conversation. Like, when we went through that conversation, then my mother was saying, "Oh, everything's fine." She's always been such a hard worker, always so selfless, that she didn't want to be a burden on her children. And I was like, are you crazy? Of course, you're not a burden and of course, we are going to do all we can.

LONNIE ALI

Lonnie Ali: You never know why you are given a certain cross to bear. Sometimes you feel like you're in this fight alone, but I think that if you have a strong spiritual base, that there's always going to be a higher being there to support you and that you can always turn to.

It's been a very important thing in my life, and in my husband's life, and I don't want to be preachy, but it is just a part of our life; and I think that it is almost a foundation in the lives of many caregivers.

You have to realize that we're all here for a reason, even in your role as a caregiver. It's keeping that positive attitude and not letting it get you down, because you never know when you may be the example for someone else; and what you're doing may not just help yourself, but thousands of others.

My husband felt that way and I'm sure Michael J. Fox felt that way in his fight for Parkinson's research; and because of their celebrity, they've been able to garner a lot of money for research—not only from Congress, but from private, individual, philanthropic donations.

So, you never know why you have something, and my husband's attitude has been, "I work with the cards dealt me, but I don't let it define who I am, and I don't let it stop me from doing what I want to do and what I need to do."

LEE WOODRUFF

Gary Barg: How did humor get you through those early days right after Bob was injured?

Lee Woodruff: We laughed. We had lots of jokes and we called him "Half head." He would struggle for words and at certain times we would laugh about some of those words. Towels were "cuddles" and thumbs were "dunkles" and he just had a whole host of things when he couldn't come up with the word in the early days. He would make the word up himself and we just learned to laugh about that.

Gary Barg: What one piece of advice would you like to leave other family caregivers with?

Lee Woodruff: One of the best pieces of advice I got was from a very dear friend who told me, "You are going to be overwhelmed with people asking you what they can do for you in the beginning. Initially, there is nothing they can do; but what you need to do is ask them to subscribe to the chit system. You say to them when they ask, "There is nothing at this moment that you can do, but can I ask you for one favor sometime in the future?"

It may be as small as asking somebody to pick up a pizza, or something larger like, "Can you spend the night with my kids because I need to be at the hospital?" Maybe it is the end, where it all becomes crazy and all you want to do is just sit by that person. You need more of your needs taken care of at that point. I would also say, "Try never to despair." I know that everybody has moments and walls or the black day that you feel is the end of the world. The truth is that each day is a new day and you can look for the little moments. Sometimes, I would just think about a great big latte with a big foamy top on it. That one little thing might be enough to put me in a good mood for that day and give me something to look forward to. I think you need to take it in bite-sized chunks when the going gets tough.

FRAN DRESCHER

Gary Barg: What advice do you have for caregivers?

Fran Drescher: I am very sympathetic to caregivers. I always acknowledge the person who is the caregiver—how hard it is for them. I always encourage them to ask for help. There have been a lot of silver linings that came out of the grief, and I think it's important that everyone finds them when you're in this situation. If you don't get something from it all, it's just such a horror without any redeeming quality. There's got to be some kind of life lesson that we can all learn from something like this when it happens—something about ourselves that can help us in our own lives.

I think that the caregiver needs as much caregiving to them as they are giving to someone else. There's nothing left when you're holding someone up from drowning. There's nothing left for you. You need people who can help you.

PARTNERING WITH THE CARE TEAM

I will fearlessly learn all I can about my loved one's healthcare needs and become an integral member of his or her medical care team.

PARTNERING WITH THE CARE TEAM

Your Care Advocates

During the first annual Fayetteville Fearless Caregiver Conference in North Carolina, we were blessed to have Kareem Strong, the Regional Ombudsman, on the expert Question and Answer panel. If you don't know what an ombudsman is, you should.

According to The National Long-Term Care Ombudsman Center, *Long-Term Care ombudsmen are advocates for residents of nursing homes, board and care homes and assisted living facilities. Ombudsmen provide information about how to find a facility and what to do to get quality care. They are trained to resolve problems. If you want, the ombudsman can assist you with complaints.*

At the event, the interaction between the attendees and the panelists were just what I love to see. Lots of questions and answers flowing in both directions. The first moment occurred when the ombudsman stated that he has an *In Case I Go Missing* file. This refers to a packet of information that he would want loved ones to find if anything were to happen to him. I wish we had such a file when my dad took ill suddenly in the early nineties. We couldn't go to him to find out things such as which bills needed to be paid and when and even where the insurance papers were located, as he was not responsive for a while. He explained that it is not necessary to give anyone your bank account password or any such personal materials. Just let them know who to call or where the necessary paperwork can be found.

I couldn't wait to get home to create my own *In Case I Go Missing* file.

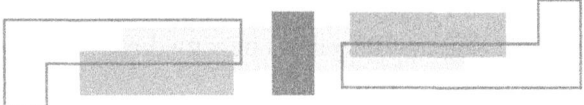

Calling Doctor Caregiver

I like to say that our work as hosts of the Fearless Caregiver conferences is to help professionalize the family caregiver and at the same time, humanize the system.

A recent event started on a high note when a doctor on the Expert Question and Answer panel asked the attendees what they want to hear from the medical professionals when they suggest that your loved one needs long-term care placement. Wow, did that open up a terrific conversation thread between caregiver and panelists.

A few interesting answers received by the doctor:
- I would like you to let me know that placement is the best solutions for my loved ones
- I want to make sure they maintain their dignity
- I would like the doctor to see us all as a team, patient (if possible) children and medical staff

We also heard this from a military veteran's spouse, "As a caregiver, I want to know the care team will really care for my husband. If you want me as a client, you better have some direct answers to my questions, because I'm trusting you with someone I love."

On another note, this caregiver spoke of some challenges she faced partnering with her husband's doctors as an active and (let's say) Fearless Caregiver, "My husband's care needs are transitioning, and I, of course, had a lot of questions for his doctors about that and about his new medication regime."

And in response to her asking questions, this fearless and formidable caregiver heard these comments from her loved one's doctors, "Are you trying to be a doctor or something? You don't need to know how this all works, just follow our instructions or call the pharmacist. " To the last comment, she responded. "Yes, but, if my husband is having a problem at 2am, and the pharmacy is already closed, what should I do?"

She went on to say that she did not think, on a whole, the medical professionals are bad or do not care for her or her husband, but it would really be nice if they knew more about her role as their patient's caregiver and wishes that they would be taught courses in medical school about what to do or say when the family caregivers ask certain questions.

My advice: if you ever get into the same situation, when the medical professional asks "what, are you trying to be a doctor?" You might consider responding that although you may not be the doctor – you are, actually, the real boss of your loved ones care, as the CEO of Caring for My Loved One, Inc. and you can make the decision of which healthcare partners to utilize.

And, by the way, you might want even to add the following phrase to your conversation: I am a Fearless Caregiver, don't mess with me!

66.7 Million Pieces of the Puzzle

Since 1995, at over 300 conferences, seminars and keynote sessions, one thing remains constant. When caregivers get the opportunity to share with one another, the wisdom is rampant. Each family caregiver has learned at least one piece of the caregiving puzzle that other caregivers are seeking.

- Need to know how to get your loved one to accept home care? **Ask a caregiver.**
- Need to know best options to stop someone from driving? **Ask a caregiver.**
- Need to know how to partner with your loved one's care team? **Ask a caregiver.**
- Need to know how to always get your fellow family members to help (well, let's not go overboard!), yet, if you want some excellent tips to help in many of these instances? **Ask a caregiver.**

Don't believe me about where caregiving wisdom is to be found? I'll prove it to you. The next time you are in a pharmacy line, hospital emergency or doctor's waiting room and you find yourself near another caregiver, take a moment to introduce yourself and share a tip about something that helps you get through the day. Then ask what gets them through their day. I think you'll be surprised how much you learn from your fellow caregiver and even more surprised about what you will teach them.

Oh, the number in the title of this article refers to how many family caregivers are in the United States today. So, to paraphrase a line used in many movies: we are not alone!

Powerful Partnerships
Prevent Painful Pitfalls

I met Tina and Tim in Tampa (okay, not their real names, but I did meet them in Tampa). They had seen me on a local call-in TV show and learned I would be speaking at a health expo that day. When I met them at the expo, I was taken by their story. For many years, they had put their lives on hold as Tina's mom, who had suddenly taken ill, moved into the guest bedroom. They did their darndest to help her and when she passed seven years later, they made plans to travel and start a new business. Unfortunately, that is when they received the call that Tim's mother had suffered a stroke.

Since both the Turners were the only children of their parents, the guest room once again became occupied. By the time I entered the story, they had the look of people who were in an emotional spiral from which they could not recover. As I spoke with them, I learned that although they had created quite a formidable team between the two of them, they never reached out to any community organization for help. They were, in fact, quite surprised to hear me answering questions from other caregivers on the show, since they thought they were the only people going through the challenges that faced them.

I also realized that even though they were extremely smart, capable and loving people, since they assumed they were the only ones going through caregiving, they never even spoke of their personal travails to their loved ones' physicians. In fact, though they were quite frugal, they didn't ever look to see if there were any choices when it came to their loved ones' services, medications and incontinence supplies and just ran into whatever store was open and grabbed whatever was on the shelves at any price. Quite an expensive oversight.

If you think that this is a situation that is unique to Tim and Tina Turner (ok, settle down), think again. Since I met them many years ago, I have seen that look in the eyes of others caught up in the same spiral. As a couple, they simply hunkered down to get the job done and had only recently realized they were in trouble. I walked them around the expo, introducing them to the appropriate care agencies, and even showed them that there were better options available for the many supplies they needed as caregivers, right under their own noses. I kept my fingers crossed.

They called me a year later. They had started going to a support group, found a physician with whom they could partner and created a cost efficiency plan for the purchase of the supplies they needed as caregivers. And most of all, they were planning their first trip away together in almost a decade. Hey, who said that TV is bad for you?

A Pleasant Surprise

I received a call this week from a gentleman who attended a Fearless Caregiver conference in Phoenix a few years ago. He is a dedicated caregiver for his wife who is living with Alzheimer's disease and wanted to talk with me about the clinical trial in which she had been enrolled.

I always say that if you want to find a real expert about any disease or illness, find a caregiver. In the few short years since we last spoke, he had become as knowledgeable as anyone I had ever spoken with about clinical trials and Alzheimer's clinical trials.

His "education by fire" didn't surprise me, he even told me of times when he was able to share new information with his wife's physicians - also not surprising. What he did say that caught me by surprise, was truly motivating. When I asked if he was caring for himself as he cared for his wife, he said "Why, of course". "In fact," he continued, "my doctor tells me that he has never seen me in as good a shape as I am in now." When I responded that I found his comment to be a pleasant surprise, he stated quite matter-of-factly, "Well, if I don't take care of myself, how can I be any help to my wife?"

Now that's music to my ears.

When the Question is the Answer

Question: what is the most important skill you need as a fearless and formidable caregiver? I know some will say it is the ability to communicate your needs with your loved ones, and honestly – that's a good answer, but, that's not it. Some would say that it is the ability to build your own personal care team from friends and family members in order to receive the care you and your love ones deserve, that's a great one, but that's not it.

Some would even say (to which I wholeheartedly agree) it is the ability to find the time to care for yourself within the whirlwind that is caregiving, and we all know how important that is for family caregivers. An important answer, indeed, but that's not it.

No, I think the most important skill we need as fearless and formidable family caregivers is the ability to ask questions. You may say "What?" And I would reply, "Exactly, nice job."

It is imperative to be able to ask any question of any member of your loved one's care team without feeling afraid that they would think less of you for not already knowing the answer you seek. So many times, our entry into the world of healthcare comes with a phone call in the middle of the night; dad has fallen, the test results have come back, and they are not good or even that our loved one has been in an accident. Our world is instantly turned upside down, our plans shattered and suddenly we need to immediately become "CEO's of our Loved Ones Care." We have entered a world chock-filled with unfamiliar acronyms; HMO, PPO, ACA, DME, LMNOP, with healthcare professionals looking to us to make life and death decisions for our loved ones.

I truly believe that the best tools at our disposal at these times are the ability to stay calm (or at least, remembering to count to ten before speaking) and the ability to ask questions of everyone involved.

The Fearless Caregiver Conferences are, as we tell our speakers, the No PowerPoint, no speechifying and no pontification zones. We and the expert speakers are certainly in the room to teach and answer questions posed by our caregiving attendees, but, most important of all, we are there to help caregivers learn how valuable it is to ask their questions.

At the events we have a moment we like to call the Question Tsunami. When we ask for questions of the attendees – it takes a while for the first hand to raise. After that question is answered, with more times than not, three or four caregivers in attendance responding with brilliant answers from their own experiences, as well as the answers given by the experts. Then a sea of hands are raised as people think of the most important question they hadn't yet asked anyone about their own caregiving.

Asking questions? Now that's the answer.

The Seven D's

Every year as the new conference season ramps up, I very much look forward to visiting with the caregivers who will be in attendance. It is always an extra special joy, however, to share the day with the grandparent caregivers in the communities in which we hold the events. These folks always enliven each Fearless Caregiver Conference and I am honored by their attendance.

So many times, the causes for grandparent caregiving are attributed to what I call the Seven Ds—Death, Disease, Divorce, Disinterest, Depression, Dollars and Drugs. These past years have seen a marked rise in grandparents acting as parents across the board. Often, they are the first safety net for children who are abandoned and whose parents are deemed unfit due to drugs, alcohol, violence or mental illness. So often, the moms and dads of these kids aren't much more than babies themselves.

The AARP saw the trend as significant enough that it founded the Grandparent Information Center in 1993 to assist these caregivers, especially those in "skipped-generation" households where a grandparent is raising a grandchild with no parent in the home. Not only are they frequently dealing with a spouse, a parent or even their own healthcare challenges; but, worst of all, they are expected to fit into those elementary school desks once again for the parent-teacher meetings!

Seriously though, the statistics are not encouraging. In a study appearing in the journal, *Archives of Pediatrics & Adolescent Medicine,* grandparent and other kinship caregivers were less than half as likely as foster caregivers to receive any type of financial support, about four times less likely to receive any form of parent training, and seven times less likely to have peer support groups or respite care.

"Our findings indicate that kinship caregivers need greater support services," the researchers wrote in a news release from the publisher. "These findings suggest that increased supervision and monitoring of the kinship environment and increased caregiver support services are urgently needed to improve outcomes of children in kinship care," they added.

So, for those grandparent and kinship caregivers, we salute you and thank you for what you are doing for your loved ones. Now, follow your own advice and have some chocolate milk and take a nap. You deserve it.

More Flies with Honey

Four flights, 3 hours of driving and a bit chillier weather than this south Floridian is used to, but the trip was more than worth the effort, as I got to spend a day with a large group of enthusiastic Oshkoshians at the Oshkosh Fearless Caregiver Conference. As usual, I am truly grateful for all I learned from the attendees.

As is my custom, I started the event by thanking four caregivers in the room for writing my next four weeks' worth of newsletters. Not that I knew who they would be at the beginning of the event, nor did I expect them to take to keyboard and produce the articles (darn!) but the wisdom shared by attendees is always so amazing, that I can usually count on at least that many articles from the day. And Oshkosh did not let me down!

First among them is the young lady who gave a memorable response to my comment that there are three words you need to have at the ready whenever you're dealing with the system (healthcare, financial, government) and they are, "Who's Your Supervisor?" As soon as I said that, she raised her hand and described how she has gotten a lot of mileage out of these words, but then added her own personal twist. She will say something like, "I thank you for your kindness and know you are doing all you can to help me and my mother. So that I can help you help us, please tell me who is your supervisor?"

I was floored, she did all the right things: treating the person on the other side of the phone with kindness, yet still getting the information she needs. She said it always works. A caregiving iron fist in a velvet glove!

Now, that's an Oshkosh trip well taken, B'Gosh!

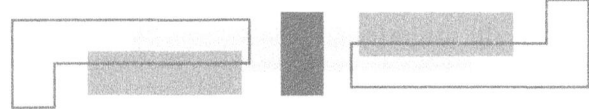

Dropping the Pins

I saw an old friend at a Boca Raton, Florida conference. I hadn't seen her for a long time and asked how she was doing. She told the attendees a story about caring for her dad that was almost an exact duplicate of a story from a caregiver at one of the first specifically rural Fearless Caregiver events. The event had been held in Arkansas and the room was packed with caregivers who had driven in from miles and miles around to be there. The questions were open, honest and wide-ranging. Yet, I had no way of being prepared for what I was about to hear as I reached a shyly waving lady with my microphone. "I was just wondering if anyone can tell me what to do. My husband has Alzheimer's disease and owns an extensive collection of guns and knives. I cannot seem to get him to stop carrying his loaded guns around the house."

You could have heard a pin drop after she stopped talking; but within minutes, she was receiving a pocketful of valuable advice, including a commitment from an elder care attorney to take on her case Pro Bono that very day. The only difference between the story the caregiver told in rural Arkansas and the one I heard in Fort Lauderdale was that the access to resources for my urban friend was greater than for the family caregiver in Arkansas. Yet, they were both able to find solutions to their challenges by reaching out to their fellow caregivers and asking for advice.

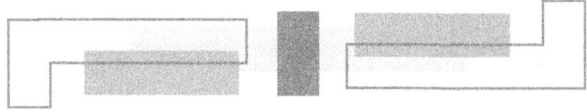

Funny Stuff

Let's talk about something that many who are not family caregivers do not understand—caregiver humor. This refers to those situations which arise out of your caregiving about which you cannot help but chuckle. A little humor can go a long way.

One of my favorite humorous stories about family caregiving came from a social worker named Claire who attended a Fearless Caregiver Conference in Wisconsin. She told a story about her days as a social work student when she was working at a long-term care facility. This was before Naomi Feil developed Validation Therapy, which encourages validating the beliefs of those living with mild dementia (as long as they are not harmful to themselves or others). In other words, communicating with them in a way that acknowledges their words and actions with respect and empathy as opposed to arguing with them.

In this case, our intrepid social worker in training was told by her superior to approach a resident who would stand in the corner for hours talking with her husband Harry. The only problem was that Harry had passed away ten years earlier. The supervisor wanted Claire to make Mrs. Smith understand that Harry was not there. Claire didn't want to do it, but she approached Mrs. Smith and told her in no uncertain terms that Harry was indeed dead. Mrs. Smith nodded in acknowledgement and then turned to her right and stated, "You hear that Harry? She says you're dead!"

It also helps when your loved one has a sense of humor as well, as witnessed in this story from my friend, Arthur Cohen:

I remember when my dad was in his last days at home, it took three of us to help transfer him from his wheelchair to his hospital bed. What made it even more difficult was the catheter, which was always uncomfortable. We accidentally tugged on it and he screamed in pain, even with the morphine. We were mortified that we hurt him, and we were trying so hard to be gentle. There was silence.

My dad, sensing our pain, said in a very matter-of-fact way, "Do I need to have this catheter forever, or just while I'm still alive?"

These stories were told many years ago and I'm still laughing...

Elevators, Planes and Arkansans

After a brief time with my feet firmly planted on good ole' Mother Earth, I am finding myself flying the friendly (!?) skies more often these days. That is the bad news, the good news is what awaits me when I land. I have been talking to so many of my personal heroes (family and professional caregivers) across the nation that I say bring on the stale coffee, hard seats and multiple concourse sprints – it's all worth it.

I was in Hot Springs and Little Rock, Arkansas to host Fearless Caregiver events a few years ago and it was my privilege to also spend a day with some truly dedicated community leaders, at the Alzheimer's Arkansas Board of Directors meeting.

In our discussions, it became obvious that one of the most important jobs these board members could have is to become Alzheimer's Arkansas Ambassadors, sharing their mission with all those they meet during their busy lives. I made sure that everyone walked away from the session with their personal inspirational ambassador "Elevator Speech." Which is to say, a heartfelt and effective statement they can share with people they may meet throughout the day about the importance of the organization that takes no longer to say than a short elevator ride.

I also think it is vitally important for us as family caregivers to develop our own short "Fearless Caregiver Elevator Speech" whenever we are dealing with the healthcare system. This is because I feel that one of our main jobs is to put a human face to our loved ones with everyone we meet along the way. When your mom or dad is in any care facility, hospital or rehab, it is our job to make sure that the staff sees your mom as Penny from Peoria who painted lovely petunias, or Sally from Secaucus who loves to sing or even sees your dad as Tom from Toronto who can still dance a mean tango, as opposed to the patient in bed 201-B window.

It is good for you, for your loved one and even for the care professionals working with them.

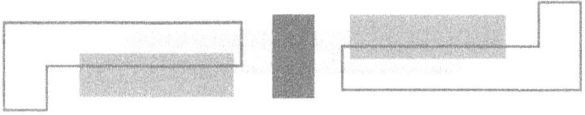

Celebrity Caregiver Wisdom

OLYMPIA DUKAKIS

Gary Barg: We always say that the caregiver should become a member of the loved one's care team. Caregivers must be able to provide information to other members of the team and be heard and be respected for it.

Olympia Dukakis: I always say that whenever a person gets sick they need advocates because it's very hard when you are dealing with the fear and the pain, and all the options and all the side effects. So you really need one or even two advocates. My husband has been very ill and I had to be his advocate, challenging this doctor and that medicine. I felt it was important because he was frightened. He had a brain aneurism. The person who is ill often can't think. He or she can't even figure out what's the next thing to do for themselves. So, somebody has to be around, and I think that caregivers are the ones who can do that.

Gary Barg: What advice would you like to share with family caregivers?

Olympia Dukakis: The hardest thing to do is acknowledge the sickness and avoid denial. Focus on today rather than on mortality. Figure out what you can do today and do it. You do have a choice regarding where things are going. I think you have to do that and plan.

PATRICIA RICHARDSON

Patricia Richardson: One of the things I learned, and that I would tell caregivers, is if you have a family member in a nursing home, never visit the same time of day. Show up at 6:00 in the morning. Show up at 8:00 at night. Never let them know when you are coming. You have to stay on top of them. And make sure you are checking all over their bodies to be sure they do not have sores. If there is ever an incident, check their chart to be sure it is notated. Make sure that there was an incident report. Facilities are supposed to be reporting if there is any kind of incident. If it is not in there, you raise Cain. I had to learn these lessons the hard way.

Gary Barg: The result is that you raised the visibility of your dad from being the patient in room 201 to being someone that people are really looking in on and caring about.

Patricia Richardson: Yes, that is the thing. Most of the nurses really mean well. You want to have a good relationship with them and treat them with the respect they deserve, but it is like a two-handed thing. On the one hand, you want to treat them with respect and have a good relationship. On the other hand, do not count on anything.

Gary Barg: You mean you should trust, but verify, and it is a partnership. You cannot immediately assume everyone is going to be terrible, but you cannot immediately assume that you are going to get the best care the system has to offer.

GAIL SHEEHY

Gary Barg: You mentioned in your book, Passages in Caregiving that we need to find a medical quarterback and I thought that is great. Could you go into that a little bit?

Gail Sheehy: Yes. What I learned was that the most important thing is to find a doctor you trust who seems to have the largest perspective. Then ask that doctor if he or she will be your medical quarterback; take in the recommendations from everybody else and present you with a checklist of what you need to do.

Gary Barg: One other thing I find very exciting about this kind of partnering with your loved one's care team is that it makes your loved one stand out.

Gail Sheehy: I think it is amazing that you are saying we want to be part of the team. I think a huge part of successful treatment is feeling that the caregiver, patient, and health professional are working together. We will help, we will do research, we will work with you, but we want you to work with us as a collaborative team.

Gary Barg: If you were only able to give family caregivers one single piece of advice, what would that be?

Gail Sheehy: You cannot do it alone. This is not a solitary occupation. If you try to be a caregiver for a loved one through months or years, even with long periods of reprieve in between, you will eventually compromise your own health, your family relationships, your social relationships, your career or your ability to work, your financial stability, your piece of mind, and find yourself in a dead end. So, the most important advice is to acknowledge, very early on, that you are paying a major life role. And it may be the role that will color your view of yourself more than any other.

ROB LOWE

Gary Barg: What would you like families to know up front when cancer is an issue?

Rob Lowe: The number one thing is to take notes and ask questions going in. Doctors are amazing, and they saved my father's life, but remember they work for you. One thing to specifically ask is, "Am I going to be at risk for infection, and if so, should I be treated for it before we begin?" Invariably, you leave the doctor's office, you drive a mile, and then you go, "Oh, I didn't ask about..." And then you don't want to call, and when you do call, you're on hold and you feel uncomfortable.

Gary Barg: So, don't be ashamed and learn to reach out, because other people are going through this.

Rob Lowe: Oh yeah, because the old cliché is true, "Knowledge is power."

MEREDITH VIEIRA & RICHARD M. COHEN

Gary Barg: If there were only one piece of advice you could leave family caregivers with, what would that be?

Meredith Viera: I believe in taking it one day at a time and seeing it as a family affair. As much as you give, you get back. I think when you keep it in that perspective, it's much healthier for everybody involved and it makes it, in some ways, light lifting because you're not doing the lifting alone.

Richard Cohen: I guess it would be for patients and caregivers to believe in themselves. I think that people are stronger than they think they are. I wish I had a dollar for every time I've heard somebody say in any context, "Oh, I couldn't ever deal with that," or "I couldn't possibly cope with that," and I always want to turn to them and say, "How do you know? You're probably much stronger than you know. How do you know you wouldn't rise to the occasion?" I think that people sell themselves short. People have a reservoir of strength and resilience that is invisible to them. It's something that they cannot see, but it's available to them. I think that if people believe in themselves and their strength a little bit more, the rest can fall into place. Whether it's getting through a bad time or whether it's confronting a doctor, both of which can be daunting. Both are doable; people just have to believe in themselves enough.

I think that we shop for consumer items with more care than we shop for doctors and I don't think any of us should hesitate to say to a physician, who is such an ongoing important part of our lives, that this isn't working. I think that people give doctors too much power. I laugh when I hear the phrase "doctor's orders" because I don't think of anything a doctor says to me as an order; I think of it as a suggestion. I think we have to take more responsibility for our own relationships with doctors. I think people are very passive and I think the days of putting doctors on pedestals, hopefully, is coming to an end.

LARRY KING

Gary Barg: You believe that people need to partner with their doctor.

Larry King: Yes, partner with your doctor. There are some people who say they don't want to bother him or her. But that's what they are there for.

Gary Barg: People are afraid of being a bother because they think "it'll affect their loved one's care."

Larry King: You are not a bother. You should be there. You don't want to tell doctors what to do, but you have every right to be kept up to date. Ask, "What's happening?" "Why is it happening?" Second opinions are very important. Doctors can be wrong, too. You have to be proactive, and you have to be loving. And, it's very good to have a doctor who knows the emotional side, too. A hand holder is very good, as well as an upbeat doctor rather than a low-key doctor. And that's important because we are all terminal. So no doctor should ever say, "You've got a week to live." This should not be said because no one knows.

Gary Barg: Don't be afraid of firing your doctor.

Larry King: Absolutely, don't be afraid. You are the client. People are so afraid of their doctors. They don't want to tell them if they don't feel well.

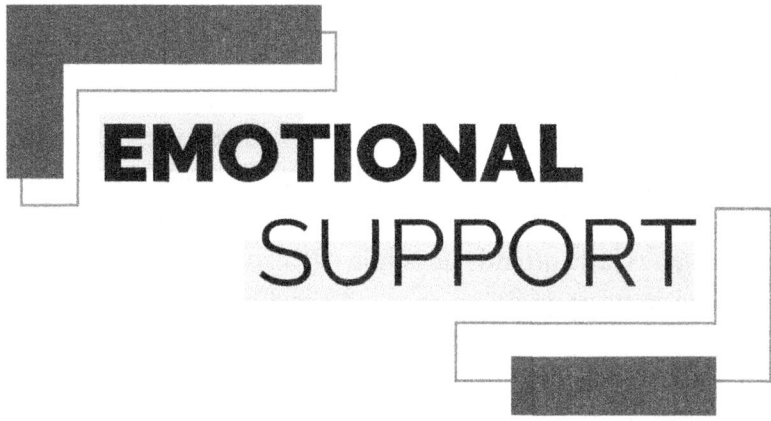
EMOTIONAL SUPPORT

I will fearlessly seek out other caregivers or care organizations and join an appropriate support group; I realize that there is strength in numbers and will not isolate myself from those who are also caring for their loved ones.

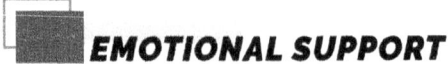

EMOTIONAL SUPPORT

"Hope Less" and "Care More"

I had the most wonderful time with my new friends in Midland, Michigan. The morning I spent with the area caregivers was full of laughter, tears and an endless flow of advice and support coming from all corners of the room.

One of the event speakers was a family caregiver, Roger, who spoke of the upcoming holiday weekend and how he worries about the care his wife June will require. He told the group that he found himself saying, "I hope she is not incontinent; I hope I can handle things; I hope we can manage." (June attends an adult day care five days a week and he starts providing care at 4:30 each morning).

When Roger spoke his anxious thoughts out loud for the first time, he began to realize that things are going to happen regardless of any of his hopes, and that he was going to be able to meet any of the challenges of her care as they came up. All he had to do is learn to "Hope Less" and "Care More."

Now that's advice we can all use, from a true caregiving expert.

Thank you, Roger.

Four P's Plus One

In each welcoming speech at our Fearless Caregiver Conferences, I always practice a bit of crystal-ball foretelling of the future. In truth, there is one single event that I can forecast will happen that day and my prediction always comes true. I start off by thanking in advance the attendee who will write my next newsletter column. Or at least they give me the idea of what to write. This event was no exception.

During the morning question and answer session, I endeavored to race around the conference room with a microphone to quickly reach the attendees as they raise their hands signaling their interest in asking a question. This is great fun and much-needed exercise (at least for me).

As the session was wrapping up a gentleman stood at the far end of my side of the room, he waved me off from bringing over the microphone stating in a booming voice, "I don't think I will need that." He was correct. He stood in response to some of the previous questions and comments from attendees about their challenges of dealing with customer service representatives by phone at various healthcare and government organizations.

His point was that when speaking with these representatives, we are the advocates for our loved ones and need to recognize ourselves as professionals. The staff members on the other end of the phone talk with many countless people every day who call in breathless, angry and unprepared to communicate their needs.

He stated that the best way to get what you need is by being:
- Prepared
- Persistent
- Professional
- Polite

I fully agree with this gentleman. If you are not confident and prepared to make your case, how can they even know where to begin to help you? Your persistence makes the difference between accepting an automatic "No" or "Sorry, it's not done that way" and getting the help you need. Your professionalism is mandatory in any caregiving situation and not to be too syrupy but "a spoon full of sugar" does go a long way in making your loved one's situation stand out from the bickering crowd.

I would make one small yet important addition to the list of P's: Pushy.

The Irony of Caregiver Guilt

After eight years of being the sole caregiver of her parents, who were both living with Alzheimer's disease, Mary had a stroke. The stroke affected her mobility and leg strength, but most importantly to Mary, it meant her caregiving days were over. Her doctor said if she went back to full-time, around-the-clock caregiving, she would likely predecease her 86- and 89-year-old parents.

Because Mary's siblings lived out of state and offered no help, long-term care placement would have to be found for her parents before she was released from the hospital. Mary's guilt about no longer being able to be the direct caregiver for her parents led to a clinical depression and affected her own rehabilitation.

In desperation, Mary contacted a therapist who helped her see that she had given her parents eight years of the best, most loving care she could, even at the expense of her own health. The therapist also pointed out that as much as Mary's parents might not like living in a long-term care facility, they would like it even less if she was institutionalized somewhere with a massive stroke, or dead because of the caregiving she provided for them. That helped ease the caregiver guilt a bit for Mary, and though she struggles with it still, there's more she can find to feel grateful about than guilty. After all, she kept both parents at home for eight years, diligently handled their finances and kept them both healthy and safe.

Regardless of the illness or disease with which your loved one is struggling, it is all too easy to find yourself in the clutches of caregiver guilt, despite the fact that you have nothing about which to feel guilty. Another thing Mary began to realize through her therapy sessions was that her guilt was slowly giving way to a different feeling – gratitude.

"I am grateful that I was given the chance to do all of this for them," Mary says now. "I'm sad it wasn't until the end of their lives, but I am grateful it was for as long as it was. Gratitude keeps me from sinking to the depths of despair over the guilt…and it also helps me put everything into perspective."

I couldn't have said it better myself.

The Fearless Caregiver's Guide to Beating Caregiver Guilt
- Recognize your feelings of caregiver guilt
- Understand the family dynamics with which you are dealing
- Learn to appreciate all you do and have done as a caregiver
- Do not feel ashamed to share your feelings
- Take the time to care for yourself

YOU are the Difference

As the height of the holiday season approached, I thought about one of my all-time favorite holiday movies, *It's a Wonderful Life*. The film's protagonist George, played to perfection by Jimmy Stewart, is disheartened about how his life had turned out and certain in the knowledge that it would make no big difference if he had never been born. Clarence, an angel seeking his wings, grants George his wish. And presto, George was never born.

The moral, of course, is that George touched so many people in his life that without him the world would be a lesser place. His existence, no matter how useless he thought it was, made a positive difference to a wide array of folks.

My point is that every time I see this movie, I think of you. Even if I don't know you personally, I do know that your existence, your heart and soul have such a profound effect on so many more people than just the loved one for whom you care.

I tell a story about some folks I know whose idea of caregiving was to swoop into town once a year, drive our mutual loved ones up to a fast food window and then just as fast as the food disappeared, so did they. It never surprised me when they would have telephonic conversations with my mom, casually explaining to her how little effort there was to this caregiving thing and asking why she was so concerned and working so hard.

I would respond to these chats with mom by explaining that there is a great lump of coal waiting for them in their psychic stockings if they did not change their ways. Furthermore, it was easy to foretell (just as Ebenezer Scrooge was warned by the Ghost of Christmas Future) exactly how their kids would be caring for them, if that time ever came.

It was, in fact, by watching my mother care for first my dad and then my grandparents; that my eyes were opened to the loving labors of family caregivers and for that my life was forever changed for the better.

So, the next time you find yourself asking "What's the difference?" please be assured that for me and for so very many people in your life...the answer to that question is *YOU* are the difference.

And just like Clarence the Angel, I can tell you with absolute certainty that you have already received your wings.

A Seat at the Table

Late last year I had the honor of speaking at the annual Focus on Caregiving Conference hosted by Mount Sinai Hospital's Wien Center on Miami Beach. It is always a great day and a true honor to be included in the lineup featuring leading physicians, social service professional and local elder attorneys. According to their website, "The Wien Center's multidisciplinary approach incorporates neurology, psychiatry, geriatrics, diagnostic imaging, counseling, social support and referral to appropriate community resources to develop successful and effective treatment options for Alzheimer's disease and other forms of dementia and memory disorders." But I know it as the place that treated my grandfather with the utmost care, diligence, professionalism and kindness, led by his physician, the world-renowned neurologist, Dr. Ranjan Duara.

At the end of my speaking session, a nattily dressed middle aged gentleman shook my hand and thanked me for my words. I thought he was a physician sitting in on the event, but in fact he told me he is a person living with Alzheimer's. He also said that he was actively and directly involved with his own treatment utilizing all the best care options prescribed by Dr. Duara. He told me that the stress his diagnosis has put on his family is his greatest motivator to work hard on his treatments and therapies. In fact, he drove himself to the event. He reminded me of my friend, the late Dr. Richard Taylor who wrote the book "Alzheimer's from the Inside Out." After his diagnosis, Richard helped form a special interest group of people living with Alzheimer's for the Alzheimer's Association, wrote a terrific weekly newsletter and traveled the world speaking to, for and about people living with Alzheimer's disease. In fact, I saw him about ten years ago speaking at the Leeza's Place in Broward County before a packed house of family caregivers. A caregiver asked Richard how she could stop her husband from repeatedly asking about their destination whenever they were to go someplace.

The exasperation she felt when relaying how she constantly answers the same question over and over within a short time span was mirrored on her face as it grew redder and redder as she spoke. Richard walked up to her and gently said "I do understand your frustration, but please remember that every single time you answered your husband's question was the very first time he remembered asking it. So instead of a simple response to a rather benign question, he would only see your increasing frustration and anger and not understand why you were in such pain."

Richard's words to the caregiver which seemed to resonate with her was "enjoy the fact that he is cognizant enough to talk with you, for someday his ability to communicate will disappear, and you will miss hearing his voice." She hugged and thanked Richard as his words resonated with her.

To truly and effectively work together against this horrible disease, all must be heard, and all voices respected.

The Boomer's Lament: or am I now they?

Speak up when we complain about how hard it is for Mom to hear; after years at the disco, no sound is too clear

Slow down when we jog by, complaining about the man with the cane, 'cause I think I just got a charley horse or at least a small sprain

When I talk with Mom's doc about her memory disorder, this time I must remember to bring a tape recorder

It's fun to watch Dad try to run a microwave; if I knew how to use my cell phone camera, that's a picture I would save

Those who are old and those who are grey, I'm glad that at least I'm nothing like they

Think about the words above when those who frustrate you are also those that you love

For it may soon be your own kids, as quick as you please, begging and pleading: "Mom, where did you hide the keys?"

Celebrity Caregiver Wisdom

LINDA DANO

Gary Barg: Were you aware of your depression during your caregiving?

Linda Dano: No. it's so interesting that you asked me that and I'll tell you why. Just last week and I was feeling sad, thinking about my dad and my mother late at night in bed looking back over my caregiving. I suddenly said, "Oh, my God, I was suffering from serious depression." Because when I was caregiving, I wouldn't talk to anybody, I didn't say what was on my mind, I didn't let anyone know I was hurting this much. I thought if I just would be quiet and not say anything, I wouldn't be a burden to the rest of my family. I'm such a believer in sharing and talking things over and not hiding things. Now I don't want anyone to be like I was when my father was ill, that I just didn't talk. Depression just comes from nowhere and it sits all over you. It's an unbelievably insidious disease that you don't even realize that you're living with. It goes to the market with you, and it goes to the dry cleaner's with you, and it goes to the dinner party with you and you don't even know it.

Gary Barg: One thing you said that I haven't really heard stated as clearly before, is that depression is a disease.

Linda Dano: How many times do you hear someone say, "Oh, I'm depressed today." It's sort of that throw-away line you hear every day when, in fact, I just wonder how many millions and millions of people walk around depressed —

severely depressed, clinically depressed — and believe that it's just part of what they're supposed to be doing. It's the way life is … It's just the way that they feel and that's that, and they don't even know that they have an illness. But they just feel sad all the time.

Gary Barg: How did your depression manifest itself?

Linda Dano: I was grieving the loss of Frank and my mom and was not sleeping. I was crying constantly, really having a rough time. Then what took over was not just the sadness and mourning and loneliness. What took over was a kind of hopelessness, a kind of "I don't care" … And every bit of passion that stands for Linda Dano was gone and I had physical pain — pain in my back, down my leg, which I couldn't understand. But you know what? That's what depression can do to you. It can absolutely alter who you are, what you are. It's an amazing illness. And scary and consuming… When the doctor said to me, "You're suffering from depression," I said, "Oh, no, you don't understand. I'm mourning my husband and mother. I just lost them both and that's what's bothering me." He said, "I know you're sad and you're very lost without them, but everything you're telling me points to depression." And you know what? He was right.

Gary Barg: What's the one most important piece of advice you would like to share with family caregivers?

Linda Dano: I want them to not shoulder all of it. They just can't … they must let others help them. If they don't, it will kill them. They must share it and ask people to help — not some of the time, but all the time. It's as simple as,

"I need to take a walk ... I'll be back in 20 minutes ..." If you try to do this caregiving on your own, I'm afraid of what can happen.

HOLLY ROBINSON PEETE & RODNEY PEETE

Gary Barg: What's the one most important piece of advice you would like to share with family caregivers?

Holly Robinson Peete: You have to take care of yourself. You cannot feel bad about giving yourself some time. You have got to have time to nurture your own soul, because if you do not, you cannot be the best caregiver. Not taking care of yourself is the worst thing that you can do. You have to give yourself a break and nurture yourself, so that you can nurture your loved one as well.

Rodney Peete: You get so consumed. I know that because not only have we been going through it, but I look at my parents who have done that for my grandmother and my grandfather and some other people in our lives. They spend all their time looking after some of the older generation and do not really take time for themselves, which makes them worn out. You have to take care of yourself healthwise and give yourself some time and give yourself a break. You are appreciated and the people that you are caring for really appreciate you. I do not think that you should ever underestimate that or think that it is not true; because even if they do not say it, you are appreciated.

ROSALYNN CARTER

Gary Barg: What's the one most important piece of advice you would like to share with family caregivers?

Rosalynn Carter: The best advice I think I can give them is to leave some time for themselves. They have to have some escape from the caregiving duties. Take some time, even if you can't get away totally.

I know one woman whose mother was sick, and couldn't get out, so she had to be taken care of all the time. Her mother wanted to see what her flowers looked like in the garden, so the woman began photographing the roses, other flowers and the trees so her mother could see the change of seasons. She got so good, she now has a photography business in her home.

Even if it's just gardening, or walking around the house, or reading a good book, people need something to take their mind off their duty. A lot of people don't like to say that they have a duty or a burden when it comes to caregiving, because there are rewards. I think that everybody feels some reward. People just need some outlet. One thing that people can do is to look up the Rosalynn Carter Institute on the Internet (www.rosalynncarter.org) and see what we're doing and send us messages for advice. People also need to know that there is help in the community, and we can help caregivers locate organizations and support groups.

LEEZA GIBBONS

Gary Barg: Really what you're saying is that isolating yourself as a caregiver doesn't help you and it doesn't help your loved one.

Leeza Gibbons: I think there's so much danger in that. Depression is obviously the byproduct of all of these diseases and if you drink, if you overeat, if you become a recluse, however it is that you manifest that, all of those things are potentially so dangerous to your own health that you can't be of any service to the one that you want to provide for.

MARLO THOMAS

Gary Barg: What would be the one most important piece of advice you would like to share with family caregivers?

Marlo Thomas: I would say to be hopeful. People cannot live without hope. Doctors can say you are going to die; doctors can say you are going to this or that, but doctors do not know everything. Nobody knows everything. There are no geniuses in this world. I think it is important to be hopeful and to notice when somebody is getting better in this little way or in that little way—to just keep feeding hope.

MONTEL WILLIAMS

Gary Barg: What would be the one most important piece of advice you would like to share with family caregivers?

Montel Williams: Caregivers have to understand that God blesses you for what you do, but if you don't stop every now and then to take care of yourself, you won't do any good for anybody. The person you're taking care of won't be able to absorb your humanity or your spirit if you're depressed, if you yourself are tired, if you aren't paying attention to your own personal health.

The one thing that I think is really important for all caregivers to understand is that every now and then, it goes back to building an honest relationship with that person; do not be afraid to speak without offending. There may come a moment when you have to tell your friend that I love you, but I need a little break, and I bet you could use a little break from me, too, so let me take one and I'll see you in a few hours or in a few days. Take a break, rather than let it fester and damage your relationship.

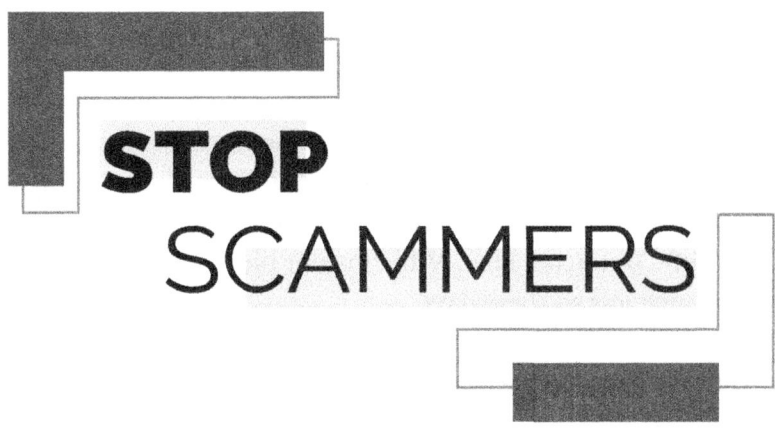

I will fearlessly not sign or approve anything I do not understand and will steadfastly request the information I need until I am satisfied with the explanations.

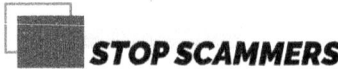 *STOP SCAMMERS*

Your Home, Your Castle, Your Wallet

Now that we are all in multiple months of sheltering-in-place, I'm sure some of our pets (talking about you, cats) would love it if we left them alone and some think this is the best thing since the invention of doggie treats (you know who you are). Another consequence for so many of us is dealing with the effects of all the extra wear and tear on our homes. This may involve the services of a contractor (plumbing, HVAC, appliance repair or replacement, etc.) Although most service providers are honest and upstanding professionals, it pays to heed the following advice as not to land in Contractor Hell. Which is not pleasant at any time but much less so these days.

Advice for dealing with contractors during Covid-19

- Check 'em out! If you don't have a provider you have worked with before, ask friends and neighbors for suggestions. Go to the Better Business Bureau and state websites to check on any complaints against their license. Ask for references
- Find out in advance what safety measures they and their staff will be employing when in your house. Masks, gloves, social distancing, etc. Pay attention to where they go in your home, so you can disinfect after they are finished.
- Make sure you and your family members are wearing masks and keep your distance while the workers are in your space. Leave the room while

they are working, if possible.
- Make sure they have a license. Many times, even if there is a license associated with the business, you never deal directly with the license holder. Make sure that the person is aware you will refer them to the proper authorities, if necessary.
- Insist on a time and payment schedule, with penalties for missed scheduled commitments and rewards for beating the schedule with competent work.
- Do not give anyone cash. Never. Not for any reason. Get receipts and when the work is done-get warranties.
- Do not pay in advance. If you are asked to pay too much before the work is done – worry.
- Watch the paperwork. Re-total figures. Ask questions. Demand proof. Demand receipts. It is your money, after all.
- "If in doubt, don't lay it out!" Get good advice from an attorney if you feel that someone may be taking advantage of you.
- Trust yourself. Don't settle for answers that don't ring true.

Now that you've passed Contractor 101, may you never have to take the final exam.

Labors of Love

As family caregivers, you are the center of the healthcare universe for your loved one. Although the great majority of professionals work very hard and care very much, it is you whose role it is to make sure that the healthcare system gives the best if has to offer to your loved one. You need to understand that many of your loved ones, especially if they do not live with you, will see a variety of doctors all of whom could unintentionally prescribe conflicting medications.

When was the last time you looked into your loved one's medicine cabinet? Have you ever scooped up all the prescription bottles into a paper bag and carried it to their pharmacist to ensure that all medications work well together? How about listing all of the prescriptions and any over the counter medications and sending the list to your loved one's primary care physician for review?

As a caregiver you also need to be adept at dealing with insurance issues. Especially in today's complicated world of HMO's, PPO's and long-term care policies. What happens if your insurer refuses to pay part, or all, of your bills? It is not that uncommon.

What many people don't realize is that they can appeal if their insurer says no. And people who know their rights have an outstanding chance of winning those appeals.

The following are a few suggestions for arming yourself should the need to appeal a denial of insurance payment arise.
- Save everything!
- Don't discard any insurance papers or any papers pertaining to your treatment.
- Save receipts for all doctor's visits and all prescriptions.
- Save copies of referrals to specialists.
- When you are speaking with any employee at the insurance company, write down their full names, positions, extensions, and whatever they tell you to do.

Keeping all these things in a portfolio can only help you organize.

Make sure your appeal is airtight. Writing a letter defining your position is your first step. A letter is documentation – a phone call is not. Your letter should be detailed, yet concise. Include important information like the claim number, group number and policy number. State the reason for coverage denial, then describe the illness and treatment. Next, state why you believe that your insurers made the wrong decision and then offer a solution. Close by saying what you would like your insurers to do. Your primary care physician and any specialists involved should write letters as well (provided they are on your side). So, don't take it lying down.

You have certain rights as an insurance consumer. A very small percentage of people ever appeal under these circumstances, but it should happen more. It is probably easier for the insurance company just to pay the claim rather than fight someone who knows how to stand up for their loved one's rights.

Phil's Dad

I heard from my friend Phil last week. He was in town for a conference and wanted to know if we could have dinner while he was here. I was happy to comply; Phil was one of my best friends when I lived in North Carolina. He was such a nice guy that some of our friends (okay, me too) had a running bet about who could tell the first story of the evening which would make Phil's eyes roll in disdain over the recounting of some recent antic. I must admit that I won more than my fair share of these contests.

We went to dinner and discussed the events of our lives which had occurred since our last meeting. Phil's parents are both still living, although his dad's recent health issues included a small stroke. Phil's dad is a retired Marine colonel who prides himself on his judgment and independence as well as his ability to read any situation and act accordingly. He had been experiencing rather severe depression since the stroke.

Phil related a development where his dad had become victim to a door-to-door sales scam to which he would previously never been prey. Among the other problems with the deal was the fact that Phil's dad signed a contract stating that the transaction took place in an office rather than at home, where it did transpire, which led to his losing some rights accorded by law. Phil's dad signed the contract on the same day as it was presented because "he did not want to be a bother" to Phil or his siblings.

It seems almost impossible that there would be that level of (saying it kindly) nefarious folks, who would spend their day trying to take advantage of our loved ones, but they are out there and they are working hard trying to profit from our pain. We must make a point of letting our loved ones know that there is no shame in telling any salesperson, "I cannot sign anything until I talked it over with my family" or better yet "…until I spoke with my attorney." This one sentence would send most of the bad guys running to the hills. Make sure that within this conversation with your loved ones, you let them know that you still respect their opinions and maybe even tell them that you want to talk over some of your personal or business decisions with them, as well.

One small suggestion: make up a card with your contact information or hand your parents a stack of your business cards instructing them to give one to whomever comes to the door looking for a signature, saying "I need to talk this over with my business partner first".

And see how fast them varmints run for the hills.

Gone Phishin'

Phishing (fish'ing) (n.)

'The act of sending an e-mail to a user falsely claiming to be an established legitimate enterprise in an attempt to scam the user into surrendering private information that will be used for identity theft. The e-mail directs the user to visit a website where they are asked to update personal information, such as passwords and credit card, social security, and bank account numbers, that the legitimate organization already has. The website, however, is bogus and set up only to steal the user's information'

I have been getting a lot of mail lately seemingly sent from well-known organizations (e.g., IRS, banks, PayPal, eBay, or a credit card issuer) telling me that I must send them my personal information immediately or dire consequences will ensue. The only problem with that is I am not a client of many of these organizations. This is what is known as *phishing*, a scam designed to part you from your hard-earned money and coveted credit. And I'm not alone in receiving these messages. As of 2014, phishing had reached over 57 million Americans compromising of at least 122 well-known brands. Phishing is also one of the very last things we need to worry about as caregivers. Of course, as in every scam, the best defense is to become an educated consumer.

The following information is presented by the Federal Trade Commission and will help you from taking the bait from these scurrilous phishing fiends:

- If you get an email or pop-up message that asks for personal or financial information, do not reply or click on the link in the message. Legitimate companies don't ask for this information via email. If you are concerned about your account, contact the organization in the email using a telephone number you know to be genuine, or open a new Internet browser session and type in the company's correct Web address. In any case, don't cut and paste the link in the message.
- Review credit card and bank account statements as soon as you receive them to determine whether there are any unauthorized charges. If your statement is late by more than a couple of days, call your credit card company or bank to confirm your billing address and account balances.
- Use anti-virus software and keep it up to date. Some phishing emails contain software that can harm your computer or track your activities on the Internet without your knowledge.
- Be cautious about opening any attachment or downloading any files from emails you receive, regardless of who sent them.
- Report suspicious activity to the FTC at www.ftc.gov/complaint, If you get spam that is phishing for information,

Game on, Fraudsters. Game on

Between phishing and Social Security scams, telemarketing fraudsters, and even sweepstake lottery scams, protecting our loved one's financial security is an ongoing battle. Unfortunately, as soon as we become aware of the enemy's strategies and find some solutions, the game changes. So, it is important for us to be ever vigilant when it comes to the ways that we and our loved ones can be fleeced (a technical term).

One way that I have found to successfully battle back this phishing tide is by actually using the internet against these fraudsters. People are becoming so savvy about not responding to internet scams that these villains are starting to resort to sending phishing letters. That's right, ink, envelope and stamps. What can be more legitimate than holding a letter in your hand? Not so fast. This is one of the times that the proper use of the internet can be of help. I have taken to the Google to research any phone number or email address connected to emails or letters asking for personal information. More times than not I can find the answers I seek by reviewing what others have reported.

Yet, sometimes even this technique can be called into question. A friend recently gave me a letter which seemed like it had been sent to him by a credit card company. He had this credit card but hadn't used it in a few years. The letter seemed official, but I went to the trusty internet search engines and found people complaining about the phone number to which my friend was asked to respond. While talking with my brother about it the next day, he immediately went to the company's official website and found the correct number listed.

Upon further review, I found out that scammers are going to the online consumer complaint sites and filling them with posts stating that the correct phone number is the scam and that, in fact, readers should call another number posted. Their number. How very helpful.

So, if it is a war between us and those that would hurt our loved ones. Game on. As any good general will tell you, it is incumbent upon us to stay in touch with the experts in the field and quickly learn to adjust our strategies, as needed.

This is a war that, as caregivers, we cannot afford to lose.

Caveat Caregiver

For thousands of years, *Caveat Emptor* has been the battle cry of all who entered the marketplace looking for goods and services and hoping for fair deals and good services. Unfortunately, this age-old phrase meaning "Let the Buyer Beware" needs a 21st century update to *Caveat Caregiver* or "Let the Caregiver Beware."

These days, so many scam artists plot to trip up our elderly loved ones or even ourselves that it is hard to keep ahead of the latest trap. Although the internet makes many things in our lives easier, our security is not one of them. Many times, our loved ones are too ashamed to tell us that they have become the victim of a scam and their silence only serves to make the situation worse. Remember that it is important to create an environment where your loved ones can feel comfortable about telling you what is happening with their finances without rebuke or scorn.

Some other Caveat Caregiver advice:

- Legitimate companies don't pressure people to act without time to investigate the deal
- Legitimate companies are glad to send information about what they're offering by mail
- Legitimate companies don't ask for cash, but con artists do because they often have trouble getting merchant approval from the credit card companies, and they also want to be hard to trace

- Legitimate companies don't ask for your Social Security number unless you are applying for credit and they need to check your credit report
- Legitimate companies only ask for financial information to bill you or debit your account for purchases you've agreed to make. Never give up your credit card number, bank account number, or other financial information when you aren't buying anything or paying with those accounts
- Legitimate companies will take "no" for an answer and will take you off their calling lists if you ask. Visit the National Do Not Call Registry (donotcall.gov) to register your phone number. If you get repeat calls, file a complaint with the registry.
- Legitimate lenders and credit card issuers do not demand payment in advance, and no one can get bad information removed from a credit file if it is accurate, no matter how much you pay them.

Identity theft is on the rise, if you feel that you have been a victim of identity theft follow the advice offered by the FTC at identitytheft.gov.

You may also want to follow another age-old piece of advice, *trust but verify*.

Celebrity Caregiver Wisdom

KERRI KASEM

Gary Barg: What's the one most important thing you'd like to share with family caregivers facing end-of-life issues?

Kerri Kasem: Get your will and estate plans in order and don't just let one person handle it. Two or three, because you never know what's going to happen to you when you get old. And it doesn't have to just be old age. You can be incapacitated through disease or through accidents. So, please, I don't care how old you are—you can be 18 years old—please have your will and estate plans in order. Even if you have nothing, at least it says this is the person I want to make decisions on my behalf. That's it. That's the most important thing.

ED ASNER

Gary Barg: I wonder if you have thought about how someone can protect themselves and their loved ones from all the scams and the frauds and the Internet crimes and identity thefts out there.

Ed Asner: Observation of an elder parent will help you find out just what is going on. Talk with them about what they are involved in. And exercise greater caution and care about checking out their mail and checking out what they are responding to and even checking out phone messages.

We do not do enough butting in on parents, within reason. I know I am so annoyed that in our family of five kids, none of us ever really sat our old man down or the old lady and asked what was it like, what did you do? And of my mother in particular: How she lived before she came from Russia and the Ukraine. We never discussed that.

HECTOR ELIZONDO

Gary Barg: If you had one piece of advice that you would like to leave family and caregivers with, what would that be?

Hector Elizondo: At the risk of sounding esoteric, we only have two real enemies in the world and that's ignorance and fear. That's it. The rest is ho-ha. There's no reason to be ignorant about the situation now. There is no reason to fear it. Get help. Simple.

YOUR LEGAL RIGHTS

I will fearlessly ensure that all of the necessary documents are in place in order for my wishes and my loved ones wishes to be met in case of a medical emergency. These will include Durable Medical Powers of Attorney, Wills, Trusts and Living Wills.

YOUR LEGAL RIGHTS

Dèjá vu

I stood in the hospital emergency room with my mother, the ER doctor and the social worker. My mother and I brought my 91-year-old grandfather in just a few hours earlier. The next few words spoken by the social worker immediately jerked me back seven years to the night my father passed away. The same hospital, the same little group: my mom, and I with two healthcare professionals and the very same question, "Does he have a living will?"

I know the implication of these words was not lost on my mother either. My dad was on his deathbed, having battled multiple myeloma for the previous year and a half. He made his wishes about his end of life decision known, but we could never actually face seeing them become real on paper. Somehow, those papers were never signed. However, I slipped a copy into my back pocket, finally realizing that perhaps we would need to face the inevitable only hours before his passing. My mother came to a similar realization. She asked me if I knew where we could find a copy of his living will. I'll never forget the expression on her face when I produced the papers on the spot. I still don't know if it was surprise or horror. Perhaps a combination of the two. She signed as my father's power of attorney and perhaps realizing that the last piece was in place for his departure, my father passed away within the hour.

So, you would think that seven years later, we, of all people, would be prepared to answer that same question.

After having created a magazine and conference series for family caregivers, after convincing people through national television and radio shows across the nation to have living wills in place for themselves and their loved ones, after being caregivers for my grandparents for the past four years, you'd think we would be prepared. You would think that we would have copies of my grandfather's living will saved in each of our cell phones. You'd think that the papers would have been signed years ago, since, not unlike my father my grandfather had also let his wishes regarding his end of life be known.

The truth is, we looked at each other as if the past seven-year gap in time was mere minutes and we suffered the same agony we suffered all those years ago. Thankfully, at that moment, we didn't need the papers, my grandfather was doing well. But, you can rest assured, they were signed soon after that night.

If I can wish anything beyond health and happiness for you and your loved ones, it is that you take the time to have your loved one's living will, healthcare surrogate and DNR (do not resuscitate) wishes legally represented. And for the sake of your loved ones, fill out these forms for yourself, as well.

Then, hopefully, all your déjà vu's will be sweet ones.

The Time is Now

When my dad became ill in 1990, I would come home to Miami to visit almost every month. But it was not until returning to Florida full-time in 1994 to help care for my grandparents that I knew what a "black hole" my mom had been living in during those past few years. She had become nurse, insurance expert, medications manager and social worker to first my dad, and then, her parents. Each day created more opportunities for fear, stress and depression.

We caregivers know a lot about fear and fearlessness. When a disease or illness enters our lives, every day becomes a struggle for the soul of our family. These battles are waged in doctor's offices, radiology waiting rooms and midnight trips to hospital emergency rooms.

What's more, we aren't alone. The latest statistics show that there are almost 70 million caregivers in the country today. So, what can you and your family do? The same as caregivers always do: stand up for your loved one's needs among your family members at the same time you advocate for him or her within the healthcare system. Acknowledge when your loved one is tired or unable to be around others for prolonged periods of time. Know what support you need from your friends and family and how to piecemeal out these responsibilities and most important of all, take care of yourself.

Do not forget to communicate with your loved one and your family members about your fears. Fear can grow to a point where it chokes your family's ability to share feelings as tensions mount. The world can all learn a lot from caregivers in these uncertain times. We have been at war with fear, grief and depression every single day as we fight for our loved one's health and well-being. We just need to remember to also fight for our own health and well-being.

Things for Caregivers to Start Doing Now

- Keep records of all medications and reactions. Make notes about what works, what doesn't and when you informed the physician of any problems
- Keep records of all doctor appointments: the reason for the visit, the doctor's responses to your concerns, any procedures performed, etc.
- Plan for the unexpected. Discuss plans and wishes of everyone involved in the caregiving family. Talk about final resting places and what arrangements your family will want
- Have an advance directive filled out and given to the primary physician and all relatives who may need the form
- Have a last will and testament completed or updated. Without a signed will, the courts will decide how to distribute the possessions of your l oved ones
- Maintain a record of where all your important documents are kept. When an emergency or tragedy occurs, locating information should not be where we spend our thoughts and energies
  When it comes to being prepared to care, there is no time like the present.

Long-Term Care - The Tool Kit

Gramp was an extraordinarily brave and hard-working man. In 1925, he jumped ship into the Boston Harbor off a Russian freighter to which he was consigned at the age of 17. Later, he made his way to New Jersey where he started a contracting company and raised a family. At the age of 35, when World War II broke out, he enlisted in the U.S. Navy.

By the early 1950's, he and his brothers owned four hotels on Miami Beach, but in the summer of 2000, he died with little money to his name in a South Florida nursing home. In only a few short years, he had depleted his significant savings maintaining his long-term care needs.

Gramp was a craftsman and he firmly believed in using the right tool for the right job. His old wooden tool kit was a world of wonder for his grandchildren. He never tired of explaining to us how each of the various tools worked and how each was best utilized.

If only Gramp had known before his illness that there was another kind of tool kit which needed to be assembled, a tool kit as important to his success as the old wooden one—a financial tool kit.

I have spent much of the last twenty-five years working to ensure that other caregiving families are not faced with financial ruin due to the increasing cost of caring for their loved ones, and that each caregiver's financial tool kit includes considering the option of long-term care coverage.

Caregivers understand what steps are needed to safeguard their loved one's physical and emotional health. We must now become adept at learning the steps needed to ensure our family's fiscal health. The lesson taught by the preceding generation and the one we must pass on to generations to come is that the tool kits you carefully assemble during your lifetime must include all instruments of preparedness to meet any situation.

Proper long-term care planning allows your loved one's financial flexibility and emotional security.

It truly is the gift of a lifetime.

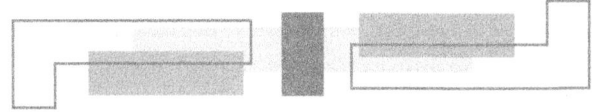

The Mal-information Tango

At a Michigan caregiving conference where I was serving as keynote speaker, a member of the expert question and answer panel which I was about to moderate approached me with a worried look on her face. She was the local representative from the Centers for Medicare and Medicaid (CMS) and she was concerned that nobody would want to ask her any questions during the session.

Although the panel was loaded with other interesting experts, from a neurologist and an eldercare attorney (always crowd pleasers) to a tremendously insightful male caregiver, I assured her that she would be an extremely effective member of the panel and had important information for this audience of family caregivers. Little did I know just how important she would become over the next hour and a half. One of the first people to raise their hands was a gentleman who related how he was planning to deal with his mother's finances in order to help her qualify for Medicare services. What he was planning raised the hairs on my neck and turned the CMS official pale as the blood rushed from her face.

For much of that session, she gamely battled misconceptions and bad advice given by caregiver's brother's, who heard it from the neighbors, who heard it from their sister's butcher's aunt's plumber's mailmen. In other words, people were not only acting upon misinformation, but what I like to call, mal-information, where what they understand to be true is not only wrong but extremely dangerous, if acted upon. With the dizzying array of potential ruinous choices that caregivers need to make on a daily basis, it is incumbent upon us to make sure that we are receiving the best possible advice, given by those in the know.

Remember, the only stupid question is the unasked question and if you find you are not satisfied with the answers you receive from anyone, keep asking until you are satisfied.

And no, taking all of mom's money out of the bank and socking it under her mattress is not such a great idea, for any reason.

NAELA all the Way

As you can well imagine, one of the most popular members of any Fearless Caregiver Conference are the attorneys. We have been blessed over the years to have local attorneys join us at the events with not only the book learning and skill set necessary, but also with plenty of heart when talking with family caregivers in need.

I always say that one of the first members on your team should be the most appropriate attorney possible. He or she can be an expert in wills and trusts and eldercare law or an expert in special needs trusts. The attorney you need is not your neighbor's brother who dabbles in real estate law. A meeting with the right lawyer for the right situation can avoid a lot of heartache down the line. This is why I would like to take a moment to introduce you to the National Academy of Elder Law Attorneys (NAELA), a professional association of attorneys dedicated to improving the quality of legal services provided to older Americans and individuals with special needs.

NAELA has established the month of May as National Elder Law Month in order to educate seniors and our families about their legal options in dealing with elder abuse and fraud, long-term and health care planning, Medicaid, Medicare, estate planning and other important issues.

All too often, we wait to deal with these issues in times of crisis, rather than working with an Elder or Special Needs Law Attorney before the crisis occurs. By planning ahead and looking to the future, seniors and people with special needs can ensure a better quality of life and that they have the services and support they need as they get older. To learn more about National Elder Law Month, visit NAELA.org.

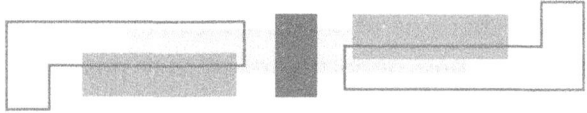

The Elder Mediation Process can bring Families Together

Steven C. Barg, Florida State Supreme Court Certified County Mediator

How do I find time to care for my mom and still work full time?
And take care of my kids?
And have a relationship with my spouse?
And not have my family members question my hard efforts?
And find money for their care?
And handle all the doctors and pharmacy visits, bill paying, home care coordination, grocery shopping and insurance follow-up?

As host of many of the Fearless Caregiver Conferences and certified by The Supreme Court of Florida as a County Civil Mediator specializing in Elder Mediation, I wanted to share this article dedicated to the many questions that are asked at a Fearless Caregiver Conference wrapped around family dynamics, family involvement and the great scope of issues that family caregivers are faced with every day.

We find that there is always a lead caregiver who, by most counts, has not been assigned the role of C.E.O. of Caring for their Loved One, but has seen the void and jumped in to help the caring process. Unfortunately, and frequently, this action is similar in nature of jumping into a rowboat filling up with water, the water representing the many tasks now taken on by the lead caregiver. My goal is to explain how to get family members to help with the overwhelming tasks and staggering amount of time that is committed to taking care of your mutual loved one. I also want to show how much easier caregiving can be when one bucket of water at a time is scooped out of the rowboat by sharing responsibilities with your family members.

I know as family members age; the family dynamics can become more entrenched and complicated. Conflicts that may have simmered below the surface for as much as decades can boil up and make family conversations very difficult. Siblings and relatives dealing with differences in their own economic and immediate family structures often find working together to help their aging parents to be challenging. Decision making as a group can seem all but impossible.

Allow me to share a few statistics from a workplace standpoint. 70% of working caregivers suffer work-related difficulties due to their role as a caregiver. (Caregiving and AARP 2015).

37% of caregivers quit their jobs or reduced their work hours to care for someone. (AARP Policy Institute).

Another set of statistics regards Baby Boomers caring for their aging parents. 80% of baby boomers reported strains on their relationship, 46% of baby boomers stated that caregiving damaged their relationship and 25% of divorced baby boomers said caregiving played a major role in their divorce. (Caring.com 2019).

Three of my dear friends wrote a book called Take Your Oxygen First: Protecting Your Health and Happiness While Caring for a Loved One with Memory Loss. Leeza Gibbons, Drs. James Huysman and Rosemary DeAngelis Laird detail how you must put the proverbial mask on yourself first to ensure you are at the fullest health and wellness before you begin helping another. So, have I encouraged you to reach out to your family to help yet?

Reaching out for family members to help may require the enlistment of an independent third party, a neutral, an Elder Mediator, who can facilitate meaningful discussion with dignity, sensitivity and respectful communication to assist families as they plan for life's changes.

A skilled elder mediator creates an atmosphere of safety and respect, listens deeply to each participant's interests and concerns, brings clarity to the issues at hand, recognizes important thoughts to discuss, and assists in exploring options. The elder mediator will create an agenda prior to the online or in person meeting with the family to help identify and develop a game plan in order for the family to move forward together. Elder Mediation provides a forum for family decision-making in a private, confidential and completely voluntary forum.

Mediators who are trained in issues related to estates, eldercare and social gerontology can help facilitate family discussions about matters relating to safety, finances and capabilities while keeping in mind the senior's desire for individual control and respect.

The ultimate goal is to develop a plan so that the proverbial boat filling up with water is slowly being bailed out with the help of other family members. Elder Mediators frequently address topics including:
- The current and future health and personal care of your loved one
- Bill paying, home upkeep and repair
- Sharing caregiving responsibilities
- Driving and transportation
- Doctor and pharmacy visits
- Insurance follow-up
- Safety and autonomy
- End of life decisions
- Health and Medical Care decisions
- Companion care and support with activities of daily living
- Financial planning and management
- Division of family possessions, heirlooms and collections
- Trusts and inheritances
- Alternative living arrangements, including independent living, assisted living and/or nursing homes

Mediation can assist siblings, relatives and aging parents to communicate more openly and directly, respect each person's dignity, and ensure that each family member's perspective is heard. As agreements are fashioned, communication skills improve, and a foundation is laid for cooperatively addressing future dilemmas.

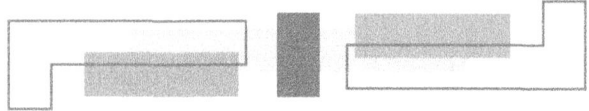

The Living Will and Coronavirus
By Jason Neufeld, Esq.

This article was written in the midst of the Coronavirus-COVID-19 quarantine madness.

As a result, health care surrogates may not be able to sign documents or communicate healthcare decisions in person. Accordingly, you may want your Health Care Surrogate and Living Will to expressly authorize healthcare surrogates to give medical directions over the phone, through Skype, Facetime or Zoom and hold medical providers harmless for relying on these non-in-person modes of communication.
The primary impact of Coronavirus, for those that contract it in its more serious form, is that it causes pneumonia and serious lung damage. Thus, your estate planning attorney or elder law attorney ought to address this specific form of artificial life sustaining treatment: Do you want to be intubated and placed on a ventilator (insertion of an endo-tracheal tube through the trachea to commence artificial breathing for a patient who cannot do so on their own).

Most standard living wills and instructions to healthcare surrogates prohibit intubation. If you contract COVID-19, and this instruction was followed, it could lead to disastrous results.

Is the Living Will Relevant to a Coronavirus Patient?

Strictly speaking, especially for those that are young that contract severe breathing difficulties due to Coronavirus, we would not expect them to be considered to be in a terminal or end stage condition (unless doctors truly believe you have no hope of recovering). But because there is a shortage of ventilators / respirators, if your living will says absolutely no ventilators or intubation, I fear that you'd be less likely to receive that potentially life-saving treatment. We honestly just don't know how medical professionals are going to interpret advanced directives, such as living wills, during a pandemic when ventilators are being rationed.

We are addressing this fear on our documents by including language that substantially says the following:

In the event that it has been determined or believed that COVID-19 is the cause of my physical or mental decline, I request that I shall be placed on a ventilator or related device until such time that a determination has been made that I have improved and such device is no longer needed - or a medical determination has been made, and my healthcare surrogate agrees, that I will not improve or survive the illness. I further request that all on or off-label medications, experimental medications, intubations, or any other therapy, treatment or effort, deemed medically prudent also be provided an utilized in an attempt to resolve my condition brought on by the Coronavirus.

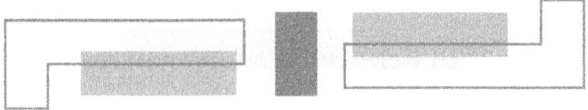

Legal Tips for Family Caregivers
Jonathan Schochor, JD

For caregivers of elderly or disabled individuals, routine and specialized medical care can be overwhelming. Communication with physicians, nurses, technicians, pharmacists and office personnel is essential to ensuring that your family member receives the best health care available. Here are several guidelines to ensure the safety and good health of those being cared for by family members.

- Keep a written log of illnesses, symptoms and medications. This list should be taken to all appointments and shared with the doctor. Do not rely on memory. Oftentimes, several doctors are treating one patient and each may not have the most recent medications, etc.
- Utilize a primary care physician who can assist with coordinating medical care. A family doctor serves as the central point of contact
- Make copies of insurance cards and claims processing information. Take this information with you to each appointment
- Obtain a power of attorney, if necessary, to provide you with the legal authority to make informed decisions regarding your loved one

Several resources are available when researching doctors and other medical providers:

The American Board of Medical Specialists (1-866-ASK-ABMS) offers a searchable database of board-certified specialists.

Consumers can check the Board of Physician Quality Assurance for disciplinary records.

Be an advocate for your loved one—ask questions, request additional information—be a part of the process.

Consider participating in a caregiver's support group. Support groups offer caregivers an opportunity to discuss their experiences in a setting that is empathetic and understanding.

Take time for yourself by asking for assistance from other family members and friends. Mental and physical exhaustion can lead to poor judgment and apathy.

Always request information pertaining to prescription medications including side effects and interactions with other medicines you or your loved one may be taking.

Five Reasons to Update Your Estate Plan: Wills, Trusts, End-of-Life Documents

Richard Barid, JD, Michael Smith, JD

As a family caregiver, we hope you are one of the 40 percent of Americans who have at least written a will or created another estate planning document.

However, even the best executed estate plan needs to be reviewed periodically to ensure that it still reflects your wishes through the many twists and turns of life.

We recommend reviewing your estate plan every three years or after any of these five life-changing events: birth or adoption, marital status change, financial change, illness or disability or death.

1) Birth or adoption: You need to update your will after the birth or adoption of a new child. A will sets out who you are, who will be in charge of settling your estate when you pass away, and how you want the things you own distributed. Anyone with minor children should have a will so they can appoint a guardian for them. Without a will, the choice of guardian is left to the courts. Once your children reach adulthood, you may omit the guardian clause.

The addition of children or grandchildren to the family may also prompt you to set up one or more trusts. A trust is a private, flexible estate planning tool that holds and distributes your assets according to a set of terms outlined in the trust. You may want a trust to fund an education or you may design a trust to incrementally distribute an inheritance based on the beneficiary's age or maturity.

2) Marital Status Change: If you have recently married, divorced or remarried, you want to make sure that your estate planning documents still reflect your wishes. Check every document that has a beneficiary designation including IRAs and life insurance policies. Unfortunately, many estate attorneys have to tell second spouses that they will not inherit as expected because their dearly beloved forgot to update the estate plan.

3) Financial Change: Financial changes, such as receiving an inheritance, may warrant a review of your estate plan. If you acquire or sell a large asset such as a house or other investment, you may want to review your estate plan. Additionally, once you reach the age of 72 you may have an IRA, 401 (k) or other qualified plan that requires distributions that may change your estate plan.

4) Illness or disability: Illness or disability in your spouse, child or other family member may cause a change to your estate plan. You may want to establish a special needs trust for a child with special needs. A special needs trust allows your child to preserve assets to improve quality of life without disqualifying him or her from Supplemental Security Income or Medicaid. If you are caring for an aging parent, you may want to establish a trust that will ensure care continues if something happens to you.

An illness or disability also may prompt you to add a power of attorney or an advance directive for healthcare to your estate plan. A durable power of attorney gives someone legal authority to make financial decisions on another's behalf. Similarly, an advance directive appoints someone to make medical treatment decisions on your behalf.

5) Death: A death of a spouse, child, grandchild or other family member may require a change to your will or trust. Also, if the person you've chosen as your child's guardian or your personal representative/executor passes away or becomes ill or disabled, you may need to alter your estate plan.

If three years have passed since you wrote or reviewed your estate plan or if any of these five life-changing events have occurred, we recommend that you review your plan with a trusted estate planning attorney to make sure your plan still reflects your life.

How to Legally Protect Your Aging Loved One
by Terry Abrams Berger, Esq.

Without proper legal planning, caring for aging loved ones is often emotionally and financially distressing for everyone involved. Families struggle at the last minute to find information, guidance and assistance to handle complex health care, financial and legal needs.

By planning ahead and obtaining the right legal documents, families can help their aging relatives gain security, take advantage of public benefits, and preserve their assets.

First, estate plans are key. They can help families avoid probate, which occurs when an individual owns assets in his or her name alone, and the court determines distribution. If not handled properly, probate can be time-consuming and costly while providing no privacy for the family.

Estate plans include wills or trusts, durable powers of attorney, health-care surrogate designations, and living wills. These documents enable individuals to manage their assets during their lifetime and upon incapacity, as well as after their death. Planning can help minimize or avoid estate taxes and ensure the senior – not the state – retains control of his or her assets.

If nothing else is done, individuals should obtain advance directives. These documents help ensure their wishes are carried out (financially and medically) in the event of their incapacity.

Advance directives include:

- **Living Will:** Documents an individual's wishes concerning prolonging life through artificial means when there is no other hope of recovery
- **Health-Care Surrogate:** Grants an individual's designee the power to access medical information otherwise prohibited by HIPAA
- **Durable Power of Attorney:** Gives an individual the power to direct the giving of gifts, apply for Medicaid, pay expenses, access retirement benefits and sell real estate.

Without these documents, a guardianship will likely be required. In addition to being costly, guardianships enable the judges – not the family members – to make critical decisions. In addition, guardianship courts hesitate to "gift away" a ward's assets for medical planning.

Families should work with trusted legal experts with experience handling elder law issues. Obtaining the right legal documents can eliminate the stress of caring for aging loved ones and give families a priceless asset: peace of mind.

Tips to Remember when Dealing with Legal Issues:

- Find an appropriate lawyer who can help you establish a will or estate plan for your relative. A lawyer can also provide strong advice on other key developments in the life of your loved one
- Discuss with your relative important financial aspects such as the location of documents, gaining access to their banking accounts, and stepping in to take over any financial responsibilities they may have
- Look into the possibility of becoming the power of attorney for your loved one if they become incapable of caring for themselves. Often a durable power of attorney can provide better coverage instead of a simple one
- A living will can provide an end of life decision for your loved one should they become terminally ill. This pivotal paper can tell a doctor just how much or how little care the person wishes to receive
- Talk with other family members about the intentions of your relative and ask their advice should you feel unsure about any matter
- Have your attorney distribute the proper documents to the doctors, banks, and health care providers of your relative
- Understand what your loved one's insurance plan calls for in the event of hospitalization or hospice care

- Be upfront with your relative about your feelings behind the decisions you make, and allow for them to offer their advice should they be of sound mind
- Find out what financial protection is offered for your loved one when it comes to their Social Security and pension benefits
- Contact local agencies that deal with legal protection of the elderly and see what services they can provide

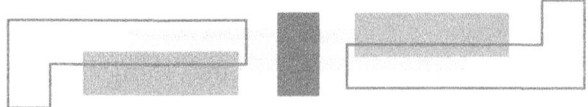

Celebrity Caregiver Wisdom

AMY GRANT

Gary Barg: Have you and your family discussed the hands-on business of caring for your loved one?

Amy Grant: My sisters Kathy and Mimi and Carol and I looked at each other and we thought, Oh my goodness! We thought the biggest gift would be to help our kids through education. Now, it is to provide for ourselves, that's just such a different message for our generation because we have not been a saving generation. But it's never too late to start working on a plan; and I think in these financial times, I don't know a family that has not worked hard to simplify. But the real elephant in the room, for all of us and for every family, is just when that shift starts. You know, when we realized that all these different things were making us scratch our heads like what are Mom and Dad doing? What did she have on when she came to the door? Why did my father make this purchase or talk to this person on the phone? Oh my gosh! We were putting out all these little fires, and then we realized that dementia was at play.

So, while they still had enough mental faculties, we went to them and said this is what we see at work. And please trust us. We need to communicate right now about what matters to you and you're going to have to trust us to carry it out. Pretty early on, we got our parents to turn over the power of attorney to my two older sisters. There were lots of conversations and lots of time spent together. All those communications are so important. We've learned so many amazing life lessons through this.

Gary Barg: There's no formula, but we can learn from other's lessons.

Amy Grant: That's true of any hard time. It is our ability to see whatever it is we're going through in a meaningful light. Otherwise, you just get trapped in why, why, why, and that's really counterproductive. I mean, tears are essential, but you just can't stay there. With my parents, I was frustrated. My mother fell again in her own home and we were going through a Rolodex of caregivers trying to find the right fit. Then a friend spoke these words to me, "Take a deep breath, Amy, and just remember this is the last great lesson your parents will teach you." That immediately created a framework for me to say, "Well, you're right. This is going to be a lesson in using my creativity, in listening to my instincts and to those moments of inspiration and direction that seem like they come out of nowhere. And trusting that, on some level, we're all led at different points in our lives when we have the greatest need." It has been an amazing journey, and I'm so grateful for it.

US SENATOR CHRIS MURPHY

Gary Barg: How do you suggest that we as family caregivers get our voice heard in the state capitals, in D.C. and even locally?

Chris Murphy: Family caregivers are stretched so thin, so many are working and then using all of their free time to provide care. Yes, I understand it's hard for caregivers to speak up politically, but there's nobody more effective to advocate on behalf of caregivers and the people that they're caring for than the caregivers themselves.

The stories that I heard from family caregivers at these round tables were so compelling that it caused me to research and introduce legislation. I think one of the simplest things to do is to organize for your local legislator a round table meeting with caregivers. I think there are a lot of members of Congress who have never really confronted this issue.

A simple thing is for a group of people who are giving care to their relative to organize a session or a meeting with their elected official, just to walk them through what their life is like and how many financial hits they have to take in order to keep their relative at home. I think just one meeting could be pretty eye-opening for a lot of elected officials.

Gary Barg: What is the most important piece of advice that you would like to share with family caregivers?

Chris Murphy: I think that there's so many decisions being made in Washington that affect their lives that if you really want to be providing care, you also have to be speaking up on behalf of caregivers. This isn't the only issue that matters here; funding for local area agencies matters as well. I think political action is difficult when you're stretched thin as a family caregiver but it's incredibly important.

WORKING WITH THE SYSTEM

I will fearlessly acknowledge when providing appropriate care for my loved one becomes impossible either because of his or her condition or my own and seek other solutions for my loved one's caregiving needs.

WORKING WITH THE SYSTEM

Choosing Well

With this decision you are not only selecting a safe and comfortable place in which your loved one will live, but also a team of healthcare professionals who will become your partners in care. Before you choose a facility, it is important to consider some important points. The first thing to remember when entering any facility is that you should trust your own senses. Are you comfortable that the facilities residents are content and well cared for in a clean and comfortable surrounding?

You may want to also:
- Conduct a "smell test." Be concerned if the facility has a strong scent of urine or even an overpowering disinfectant smell
- Speak to as many different staff and residents as possible. Get a sense of how the residents and workers feel about the facility; do they enjoy living or working there?
- Talk frankly with family members of other residents
- Notice how the staff treats the other residents in their care, that probably reflects the level of care your loved one will receive
- Visit at differing times of day and evening before making a decision
- Ask about the level of staff to resident. How many are on duty during the day, overnight and on weekends?

- Ask about the facility's policy for holding a bed if your loved one must be hospitalized or go into a rehabilitation facility for a temporary period
- Ask to see a copy of the facilities contract and read it carefully. You may want to consult with an attorney before signing a contract
- Find out if the facility has a comprehensive disaster and emergency plan including evacuation procedures and when it was last updated. Ask to review a copy of the plan

Visit a few area facilities before making a choice. You are in charge of this important decision and should never be made to feel as you were pressured to choose any particular facility. You need to research, ask plenty of questions and above all, trust your own instincts.

Sometimes, All It Takes Is Gall

Recently a small group of friends and I visited a friend of ours who was in intensive care after he experienced complications following gall bladder surgery. He was telling us about a terrible experience he had with one of the nurses caring for him in a different wing of the hospital right after his procedure. According to him, the nurse was openly hostile a few times and did not respond to his reports of the physical discomfort which was an indicator of the trauma eventually causing his trip to the ICU. He was worried about reporting the nurse to the hospital complaint line, as he would be returning to that ward within a few days and feared retribution.

One of our friends, a hospital based therapist, said that not only should he report his concerns, but also said that whenever a patient or caregiver of a patient in the hospital where she works takes notes, the staff is seen to pay specific and positive attention to that patient. That was a revelation for the rest of us in the room. For me, knowing as many dedicated care professionals as I do, I could see that the note-taking would not bother them, but as in my friend's case, it is nice to see that proactive involvement is not only nothing to fear, but would be noticed and appreciated by the majority of care professionals.

Notes on Notetaking

In an article on caregiver.com, I shared the story of my friend who was in the hospital and felt that he was mistreated by a staff member. A mutual friend who works in hospital settings suggested that he starts taking notes during his stay in the hospital, but he was concerned about being seen documenting his experiences for fear of retribution from a staff member. I heard from many caregivers about this issue and would like to share some of their comments with you:

Healthcare professionals who have nasty attitudes must be reported. They're supposed to deliver a courteous and dedicated service to their patients who are in pain. You could just imagine people suffering from physical and emotional pain and be treated that way. Caregivers must stick to their vows of attending to anyone who needs their tender and loving care. Grrr.. Grrr.. I really hate hypocrites, especially in the caregiving sectors.

Your article on notetaking hit the mark today. I took care of my mother for three years as she slowly faded away from Alzheimer's disease. At one point we were in the hospital because she had a severe nosebleed and my brothers thought I was crazy taking notes all the time. I would write down times of nurse checks while in the ER and any new doctor or intern name. As it turned out, not only did it help when she was transferred to a regular room, but months later when we had to sort out insurance claims. I had all the information I needed to cross-reference all of those "miscellaneous" tests and doctor visits on the bills. Let me tell you, my brothers were happy when we challenged a few of the procedures that I hadn't noted taking place.

Many hospitals have patient advocates who make rounds and handle patient/caregiver complaints. These dedicated professionals go by many different titles: Patient Relations, Patient Advocates, Ombudsman, Customer Service and Guest Relations, but have one purpose - to facilitate and improve the patient experience.

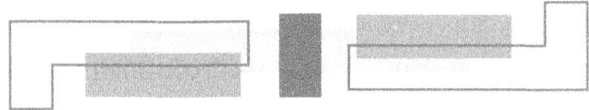

Three Little Words

The call from her brother came for Trudy in the middle of her workday. Her mom, who had been ill for a few years, had passed away. Trudy left work immediately and set out for her brother's house. This was a four-hour trip which Trudy had taken almost every weekend since her mom became ill. Trudy's brother Bob, in whose home their mom had been living, was the primary caregiver during these past few years. After the funeral, Trudy returned home only to receive another phone call from her brother's house. This time the call came from her sister-in -law. Bob had a heart attack and needed an immediate triple bypass. Trudy was on the road once again.

A few nights later, as she sat by her unconscious brother's bedside in the regional hospital, Trudy began to realize that his bed sheets had become soiled and would need to be changed. She went out to the nurse on duty, who told her that no one would be able to attend to her brother for at least an hour, when the paperwork was finished. So, Trudy returned to the room and changed his sheets by herself. When we spoke after her return home, she told me that she did not argue with the nurse because she was afraid that any disagreement would affect her brother's care. I was not too surprised, because many caregivers I talk with have the same concern, "If I am a squeaky wheel, my loved one's care will suffer".

My answer to Trudy was to respond with three little words that I have shared with attendees at Fearless Caregiver conferences for many years. I told Trudy that she needs to say these words firmly and repeatedly until she is satisfied with the results. Those three words…"Who's your supervisor?" Three other appropriate words in this situation would be to "document, document, document".

Although I would hope that any disagreement with your loved one's care staff can be handled in a calm and professional manner and I know of countless professionals who diligently work towards providing every patient the best possible care, any attempt to elicit retribution upon your loved one for your comments should be dealt with seriously, immediately and possibly even legally.

Partnering with your Loved One's Medical Professionals

I received the following email from a reader about an issue of importance to a great many of us:

> *My dad is dealing with rheumatoid arthritis, stroke recovery and prostate cancer. I do not know all the medications he is on. The doctors seemed to feel no compunction about scolding our brother that my dad was losing weight and muscle mass. What bothers me about the doctors, then, is that this is done without really knowing what he does eat, without scolding my dad for his finicky tastes, and without any of the need for exercise to prevent loss of muscle mass.*
>
> *And here's the kicker: when I ask my brother (who accompanies my dad to the doctor and has primary responsibility for the backbreaking task of caring for him, which he discharges selflessly) if he asked the doctor any practical questions about how to do this any better, he tells me he is afraid to alienate the doctor for fear of reprisal. This fear is not unfounded. In our one-horse town any such question is actually treated as some sort of challenge of their authority. It would certainly be in the best interest of their patients if the caregivers are treated like a part of a team and armed with the most comprehensive information they can use and if their practical questions are answered. If they have no answers, why do they need to pretend that the questions are inappropriate?*

LB

My Response to LB:

I think you have made some incredibly important points and I'm glad you took the time to write. First, you hit the nail on the head about communicating with doctors and family members. Your goal is to become an acknowledged member of your loved one's healthcare team. After all, they more likely than not, see him only a few times a month, while your family's knowledge of him is consistent and much deeper. You should be considered an asset to them as they evaluate his health. I know that, in many cases as you mentioned such help is not easily appreciated or sought. But the statistics are truly on our side.

Did you know that over 70% of doctors will listen to and even adjust their care when a caregiver brings them qualified and well-documented information? Understanding that you have your hands full with an entrenched medical community in a small town, (not to mention a parent who is not an active participant in his own care), making a solid case is your best bet.

- Start (or have your brother start) a journal of what your dad really eats throughout the day and his daily health, include his exercise regime (if any)
- Create a list of questions that you want the care professionals to answer
- Find some research backing up the points you want them to consider and when you are ready, make an appointment with the doctor and/or dietician with these specific communication goals in hand

In this manner, you put the ball in their court. They can not easily say that you are just an over-reactive daughter or sun when you are armed with the facts. If your dad does go into a care facility (rehab or hospital) they have care plan meetings in which you should be able to participate. What you are working against are the points that you brought up, but also the fact that your doctors are scientists and have spent many years dealing with concerned but unprepared loved ones, who do not bring these things to their attention in a manner in which they could and would respect. Let them know that you and your brother are formidable allies in your dad's care, and that you are not going to go away quietly or easily.

Your dad is lucky to have you both on his team.

Preaching to the Pews

I'd like to spend a few minutes addressing the healthcare professionals and non-profit organizational leaders reading this today. Please do not overlook your real partner in the person of your client's family caregivers, and also do not forget that these same caregivers are prone to take themselves out of the all-important Circle of Care.

Caregiving Circle of Care

- We make sure our loved ones get all the respite they need, but never give ourselves a break
- We make sure our loved ones receive the medical attention they need; yet forgo our own basic checkups

- We make sure that our loved ones get the nutrition they need, but we only eat our meals ordered through a clown's mouth from a fast food drive-through lane at midnight

Remember that family caregivers are your best in-home partner. They spend their days carrying out the instructions established for their loved one's care but in so doing they put themselves under great stress. So, celebrate them and help them give their loved ones the benefit of your wealth of knowledge, talent and experience and while you are at it, make sure to find out how they're doing, as well.

The truth is that I am probably preaching to the pews as most of the best care advocates and healthcare professionals

I have met over the years started their careers after having cared for their loved ones themselves.

It is with these facts in mind that I would like to leave you with a simple request, and that is to add one more person to the list of people for whom you care - yourself. I know how hard you work for your clients and that many of you go home at night to your own caregiving duties. We need you to be at your best as do your loved ones, so please remember that you are certainly included in the Circle of Care.

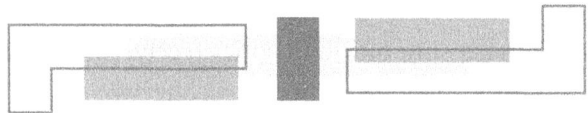

Caregiver Curmudgeon's Communication Commandments

Lest ye not suffer unto us the words "suffer," "suffering with," and (worst of all) "victim" when talking about our loved ones. For example, a person living with Alzheimer's disease also has many more facets to their existence of importance to themselves and those who love them. People do not need to be dehumanized by being categorized, classified and defined by their disease, in person or in print. The fact that our loved ones are battling these diseases or illnesses should not be their defining characteristic when writing or talking about them. (Feel free to replace the word "Alzheimer's" in the above paragraph with any other disease, illness or disorder.) I am astonished by how many experts use these phrases in their press releases, books and writings. I don't know about you, but I think we can all do better.

Honor thy father and mother as they would wish to be honored.

Even if many of the tables have turned and you are performing a lot of the duties for your own parents analogous to parenting a child, they have never stopped being your parents. How about using the phrase "Partnering with our Parents" or as in Howard Gleckman's book title *Caring for Our Parents*? Even if they cannot offer any support as we care for them, and in fact if their mental state offers specific challenges to the help we do give, I think it is imperative that they at least feel as if they are still in charge. Ask Dad's opinion about what show to watch; give Mom a basket of mismatched socks to fold when you are doing laundry. Only you know what technique might work for your loved one.

Speaketh ye with love about those whom we love.

I love to read when the people for whom we care are referred to as "loved ones" or even "clients" as opposed to "care recipients" or "patients." One should only be referred to as a patient by their own care professional (and even then, I like the word "client" better.)

As they say in elementary school, "Sticks and stones can break my bones, but words can never harm me." Perhaps, but they can stigmatize and negatively define a relationship in a way that you didn't mean for it to be defined.

Top Ten Things a Caregiver Needs from a Health Care Provider

1. **Attention:** The caregiver's loved one may be the 27th similar case you've seen today, but to the caregiver, this is Mom or Dad, Sister or Husband

2. **Compassion:** Be diligent in its application

3. **Time:** A few moments of your undivided time is some of the strongest medicine you'll ever administer -- and it costs so very little

4. **Respect:** The person pushing the wheelchair is also part-time bookkeeper, psychologist, dietitian, insurance and incontinence expert and a full time general in the war they are waging with this illness. They not only need your respect, they *DESERVE* it

5. **Dedication:** Be relentless in your devotion to your craft. The caregiver has entrusted you with their most valuable asset - their loved one. You earn that trust with your skill, knowledge base and ability

6. **Honesty:** The caregiver is your partner in this endeavor, they deserve (and can handle) the truth

7. **Prudence:** The graceful administration of the truth is a true test of a caring professional

8. **Advocacy:** Never accept less than the best your system has to offer their loved one

Working within the System

9. Understanding: The caregiver plays a pivotal role in the well-being of your patient. Understanding the needs, wishes and fears of the caregiver improves your patient's care

10. Your well-being: Know your emotional limit and learn when to ask for help. Your loved ones as well as the caregiver's loved one need you to remain well

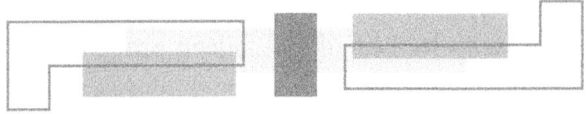

Mr. & Mrs. Smith

I was leaving the conference hall where the 22nd annual conference held by the Western Carolina Alzheimer's Association had just concluded. It was an honor to be asked to speak at the event especially since it was aptly titled, *Support for Today's Caregiver*. The event was held on a perfect fall day, crisp and clear, with a cloudless Carolina blue sky. Walking from the conference hall to the car which would take me back to the airport, I took my time to relish in the sights and smells that can only be experienced on such a day in such a place.

Walking beside me was a middle-aged couple; let's call them Dan and Jane Smith for the sake of anonymity (if not literary originality). Jane started to talk as we walked together, saying that she had liked the conference very much. She told me that when her family's loved one was diagnosed with Alzheimer's disease, the doctor told them that they were dealing with FTD and that they should come in for another appointment in four months. Later that night, convinced that he wasn't talking about the floral distribution organization, she looked up the initials and was aghast to find out that in this case FTD stood for frontotemporal dementia. To her credit, she immediately called the doctor and demanded more information, and a better bedside manner.

Dan Smith, who looked like a college professor complete with tweed jacket and wire-rimmed glasses added "I've been in education most of my life and I've noticed that the challenge of Alzheimer's disease is usually to be found in the lack of communication." Although this seems like an obvious statement for anyone with a loved one living with memory disorder to make, Dan was actually referring to the health care professionals that he has met since his own diagnosis with Alzheimer's disease two years ago.

I think we can all still learn a thing or two from Professor Smith.

PREVENTING SENIOR ACCIDENTAL OVERDOSES

A growing concern for family caregivers is the possibility of a loved one's accidental overdose. This is an issue I hear about with alarming frequency as we travel the country on our annual Fearless Caregiver Conference tours. If nothing else, the statistics bear out the potential for danger to our loved ones.

Older women consume 60 percent of all prescription and over-the-counter medications. The number of prescriptions written for older adults averages 18.5 per person per year, and 83 percent of people over 65 are taking prescription medications. With this many medications to take on a regular basis, an accidental overdose could be a problem for anyone; but for many of our loved ones, the risks are increased by memory loss, hearing difficulties and low vision.

It is vitally important that, as caregivers, we pay attention to the potential for an accidental overdose by a loved one. Some things we can do:

- Pay attention to any changes in their speech patterns, mental acuity, physical strength or level of depression or confusion
- Regularly check the medicine cabinet and refrigerator for medication usage patterns, expiration dates, and to ensure timely refills

- Scoop all the prescription bottles into a paper bag and carry them to their pharmacist to ensure that all medications work well together. It is best to use the same pharmacy for all prescriptions. One of the most important partnerships we can have with a care professional is often overlooked – the pharmacist
- Many of our loved ones are receiving medications from multiple doctors. Make a list of all the prescriptions and any over-the-counter medications they are taking and send it to your loved one's primary care physician for review

When discussing these concerns with your loved ones, remember that your most effective weapons against an accidental overdose are respect and understanding. Successful medication management works best when you are working as a team.

Today's Caregiver Family Checklist

The most loving gift a person can give to one's family is to put your affairs in order before a disaster or medical emergency. To assist in providing that gift, *Today's Caregiver Magazine* has compiled the following list. The information and documents you should have prepared:

1. All bank accounts numbers, types of accounts and the location of banks
2. Insurance Company, policy number, beneficiary as stated on the policies and type of insurance (health, life, long term care, automobile, etc.)
3. Deed and titles to ALL property
4. Loan/lien information, who holds them and if there are any death provisions
5. Social Security and Medicare numbers
6. Military history, affiliations and papers (including discharge papers)
7. Up to date will in a safe place (inform family where the Will is located)
8. Living Will or other Advanced Directive appropriate to your state of residence
9. Durable Power of Attorney
10. Instructions for funeral services and burial (if arrangements have been secured, name and location of funeral home)

Celebrity Caregiver Wisdom

BOB GOEN

Gary Barg: Can you describe your father's transition from home to a facility?

Bob Goen: We left it completely up to mom the whole time. She was shouldering the burden from the word go, so we told her that whenever you want to do it, you tell us and we'll get it done. Wow, I'll never forget the phone call that one morning when she said, " I just can't do this anymore." It was the hardest thing she ever had to do, but for us, the kids (I have two older sisters), to go along with that request was easy, because we weren't living with it on a day-to-day basis. The difficulty was the actual process of putting him in the home. That was, to this day, the hardest day of my life. That's the most painful part of this whole thing, emotionally. Taking dad's stuff and putting him in the car and having to makeup this scenario as to why he's going there, basically kind of lying to him in order to get him to just go along for a while.

Gary Barg: I call those "loving lies."

Bob Goen: They were, and it was either we lie to dad, or we watch my mom slowly die. We were already watching dad slowly die, and it was a lie that had to be told. We said to dad that mom was going off on a cruise for a couple of weeks and that I would be out of town, and Barbara and Judy, my two sisters, were going to have trouble getting away from work to watch him, so we just wanted to put him in there until mom gets back. He begrudgingly agreed, and so we went down there. I was the one in the family who was able to hold it together long enough to get him settled in his new room, to talk to him, to soothe him and to comfort him. He kept trying to leave, and I don't know where the strength came from, because I usually do not have it, but I was able to sit with him for a couple of hours, and convince him that this was the right thing to do. One-by-one, everyone else in the family left and went out into the waiting room, because they couldn't do it anymore, because they were emotionally drained. One of the most memorable moments, in a real negative way, was when I left him in his room, and walked into the waiting room, where the rest of my family was sitting. It was an extremely powerful moment when the four of us just held on to each other, and I remember my sister saying, "My God, when you turned the corner into that room, your face was a color I had never seen before." We just clung to each other.

Gary Barg: Was your mom able to start taking care of herself after your dad left home?

Bob Goen: Yeah, that was the best part, because she was able to focus on herself. She could now do the smallest things, like go to lunch, or work in the garden, talk on the phone. The slightest, nothing little pieces of the day became a huge joy to her. Eventually, she was able to go away on vacation, and go to church, and do all the little things people take for granted.

Gary Barg: What caregivers often don't realize when thinking about placing a loved one in a facility is that they are still in charge, it's just that their role changes.

Bob Goen: Mom did that; she really took charge of how the facility dealt with Dad, and she was over there two or three times a week. I'm not sure how it all evolved, but the people at this facility really embraced us as a family, because we were so unified in what we were doing. We've got a really strong bond and love each other dearly. I think they really related to that, and they appreciated it, and they loved to see the support that we gave. Mom would go over there, and it would be like the president had come to town. She was always welcomed with open arms and enthusiasm. It was the right scenario, and it made a huge difference for us.

SCOTT SIMON

Gary Barg: Talking about the reactions you got from your tweets and the people who wonder about motivation, I think there are two things. One, in a recent interview, you said that having a loved one in the hospital has moments of panic and anxiety, separated by hours of tedium. Absolutely. And two, I think that any family caregiver understands that there is so much humor in caregiving and your tweets really express that.

Scott Simon: I think in another tweet I said that people in my profession, so-called profession, journalists, tell ourselves that we are hard and cynical because of all we see in life. And ICU nurses and other personnel there see, as a generalization, more in a month than we will see in 10 years. And they just come out better, kinder, stronger, and more humorous because of it. I am just in awe of them.

Gary Barg: It is important that we see each other as human beings. That is a job role for family caregivers to take on, to make sure that they are standing in the middle of the situation and treating the professionals, when deserved, with respect and accommodation and showing them who their loved one is as an individual. And if their loved one is not able to communicate themselves, telling stories, which is what you do.

Scott Simon: I think you put your finger on something. My mother, until about the last 24 hours, was in a position to make jokes, laugh (albeit it became painful for her), and communicate. I think that is not true, obviously, of a lot of people in that position. I wanted the relatively young doctors who were working there to see the whole person, not just the person who was almost 85, who was totally having trouble and was in her last days on earth. It was important for me that they also saw her as a person; that they got some sense of the funny, lively person who was once their age and who had children and grandchildren, and had a tough and interesting life. I think that is very important in terms of making that palpable human connection between people. And I think it makes all the difference between seeing someone as a patient in a bed and seeing them as a human being.

I suspect that is something that one way or another we can all do in our individual lives and disciplines. I mean, I know that absolutely dovetails with something that I try and tell some of our young reporters. Having covered bits and pieces of 10 wars is when you begin to think you have seen it all before. That is a problem because you have not.

Gary Barg: What would be the one most important piece of information that you would like to share with family caregivers?

Scott Simon: I would say to remember the person that you are helping through life was young once and had a life different than the one that you are seeing right now. And so, as far as you can, try and get to know and take care of that person, not just the needy one who is in front of you.

MARILU HENNER

Gary Barg: At the Fearless Caregiver Conference, our main emphasis is one that I have heard you talk about before; the fact that honest, open, frank communication is key to caring for a loved one.

Marilu Henner: Absolutely. You have to use humor and sensitivity. You have to be fearless, of course. You have to not let doctors talk you out of asking questions or intimidate you so that you don't get your questions answered, because a lot of times we're so afraid to open up our mouths.

Trust me. I am not from the keep quiet and they'll let me live school. I want to make noise if noise needs to be made. You don't even have to do it in an obnoxious way. You just have to do it in a very loving but firm way, especially if you have a reluctant partner who doesn't want to make waves or feels embarrassed.

I keep saying to people, the caregiver has to be the brave one. The patient is so frightened, and they're so stuck.

Their whole life is flashing in front of them. They're just so afraid of not being who they were and who they want to become. They're afraid of people at work finding out. They're afraid of being labeled as a patient, or they feel like they're going to be alone and in the dark and not have enough information.

That's why somebody in your corner, that's brave enough to say, "Hey, I'll go with you," and cares enough about you to say, "I'll ask the questions. You can talk to me. There's nothing that's out of the realm of possibilities for us to be able to discuss." So, you've got to find that person. That's the caregiver.

The caregiver, of course, has to take care of themselves. I keep saying that one of the things I learned being a caregiver is that you have to dress warm, because hospitals and doctor's offices are always freezing cold. I learned to multi-task my health by not only layering up and making sure I was dressed warm and wore comfortable shoes, but I would also go up and down the staircases, or I'd walk around the block, or around the hospital, and I learned how to hydrate and bring healthy snacks. You just have to take care of yourself too. I think a lot of times caregivers forget to do that.

Gary Barg: What guidance would you offer other caregivers who just walked into this situation?

Marilu Henner: I would first of all analyze why you're in fear. What's your earlier experience that put you in the fearful position of not asking questions? Maybe it was a mean teacher at school, then get over it. I think if you're prepared, and you're coming off very pedantic or like a shrew or something, that's not going to get the job done. Then, if you're not only talking to the patient with a certain kindness and sensitivity in your voice, but also to the doctor having done the homework.

Gary Barg: What would be the one most important piece of information that you would like to share with family caregivers?

Marilu Henner: I would say be brave. Be brave. Be fearless. Caregivers are the brave ones who have the snowplow that everybody else gets to ski behind. So, I don't mind being the snowplow starting with my conversation with you right now.

Working within the System

The *New* New Normal

No matter how your caregiving started, from that metaphorical phone call in the middle of the night to inform you that there has been an accident, to a doctor's office consultation that changed your lives, you immediately entered the New Normal of family caregiving. Suddenly, you had to learn new terms such as palliative care, HIPPA, Advanced Directives and Ombudsman.

As we all entered the *New* New Normal as family caregivers due to the pandemic and even in its aftermath, there were additional phrases you had to learn: social distancing, telehealth, telemedicine, N-95 masks and sheltering-in-place.

Thankfully, many of the same skills you learned as a family caregiver still apply. How to navigate an unfamiliar system, stand up for your loved one's care and even remain fearless throughout uncertainty. Yet, something that remains constant is the fact that these journeys are better when traveled together. One of the challenges that we face as family caregivers while not being able to spend time with one another is that it is harder to share the lessons learned from our fellow caregivers.

My greatest joy of hosting the Fearless Caregiver Conferences is to hear attendees share their most vexing questions only to receive a multitude of truly insightful answers from their fellow attendees who have already solved that piece of the caregiving puzzle for themselves. It is my pleasure to be able to share some of these caregiving puzzle pieces from the over 100,000 family caregivers who have joined us at the events since 1998.

Although, we also support caregivers through Today's Caregiver magazine (website, newsletters and podcast), our social media outreach and even with webinars and videos, I very much look forward to once again spending time with you in your own communities.

Stay well, safe and most of all…Fearless.

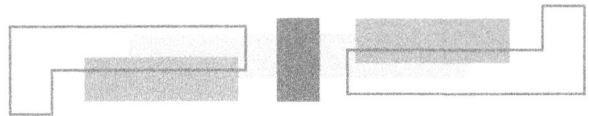

Special Thanks

The Living Will and Coronavirus
By Jason Neufeld, Esq. Elder Needs Law, PLLC
elderneedslaw.com

Legal Tips for Family Caregivers
By Jonathan Schochor, JD
Schochor, Federico and Staton, P.A.
sfspa.com

Five Reasons to Update Your Estate Plan: Wills, Trusts End-of-Life Documents
By Richard Barid, JD, Michael Smith, JD
smithbarid.com

How to Legally Protect Your Aging Loved One
By Terry Abrams Berger, Esq.
bergerlaw-llc.com